# 2000 Rx

## BREAKTHROUGHS IN HEALTH, MEDICINE, AND LONGEVITY BY THE YEAR 2000 AND BEYOND

## Jeffrey A. Fisher, M.D.

SIMON & SCHUSTER
New York London Toronto Sydney Tokyo Singapore

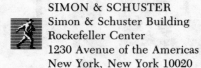

SIMON & SCHUSTER
Simon & Schuster Building
Rockefeller Center
1230 Avenue of the Americas
New York, New York 10020

Designed by Carla Weise/Levavi & Levavi
Manufactured in the United States of America

10   9   8   7   6   5   4   3   2   1

Library of Congress Cataloging-in-Publication Data

Fisher, Jeffrey A., date
     Rx2000 : breakthroughs in health, medicine, and longevity
by the year 2000 and beyond / Jeffrey A. Fisher.
          p.     cm.
     Includes bibliographical references and index.
     1. Medical innovations.   I. Title.   II.. Title: Breakthroughs
in health, medicine, and longevity by the year 2000 and beyond.
     [DNLM: 1. Delivery of Health Care—trends. 2 Forecasting.
3. Technology, Medical—trends.   W 84.1 F534r]
     R855.3.F57   1992
     610'.9'0501—dc20
     DNLM/DLC
     for Library of Congress                                   92-9668
                                                                CIP

ISBN: 0-671-73844-5

*For my children:*
Brett, Ben and Erin

# Contents

—— **PART III:** MAJOR ILLNESSES AND MINOR ——
CONDITIONS  133

# Scientific Acknowledgments

THIS BOOK IS, IN THE TRUEST SENSE, A COLLABORATION WITH A long list of medical and scientific experts who were willing to share with me their thoughts, hopes, anxieties and predictions. They gave me their time, in many instances admitted me to their research laboratories and frequently showed courage in making their vision of the future known to me.

I recorded their views, read their papers and sometimes looked over their shoulder while they worked. I could not have written this book without them. I thank them for their enormous generosity.

Armed with their insights, and much additional research on my own, I have created a picture of the future that in some instances may seem like science fiction, but none of it is. Everything you read in this book is going to happen. How it will happen and when it will happen may vary somewhat from the scenarios you're about to read, but I have written the most scientifically accurate view of the future I could, based on years of intensive probing and the wisdom of the following men and women:

Thomas Alt, M.D.—President, American College of Cosmetic Surgeons; Minneapolis, MN

Julius Axelrod, Ph.D.—National Institute of Mental Health, Bethesda, MD; Nobel Laureate in Medicine and Physiology, 1970

Arthur Balin, M.D., Ph.D.— President, American Aging Association; Philadelphia, PA

Herbert Benson, M.D.—Professor of Medicine, Harvard Medical School; Director, Mind/Body Institute, Boston, MA

Jean Bernard, M.D.—Président du Comite Consultatif National d'Éthique des Sciences de la vie et de la santé, Paris, France

Jan Breslow, M.D.—Director, Laboratory of Biochemical Genetics and Metabolism, Rockefeller University, New York, NY

Craig Brod, Ph.D.—Psychotherapist, Oakland, CA; author of *Technostress*

Aldo Campana, M.D.—Professor of Obstetrics and Gynecology, Geneva University School of Medicine, Geneva, Switzerland; former President, Swiss Society of Fertility

Arthur Caplan, Ph.D.—Director, Center for Biomedical Ethics, Professor of Surgery and Philosophy, University of Minnesota Medical Center, Minneapolis, MN

William Castelli, M.D.—Medical Director, Framingham Heart Study, Framingham, MA

Peter Cerutti, M.D., Ph.D.—Director of Carcinogenesis, Swiss Institute for Experimental Cancer Research, Lausanne, Switzerland

Kenneth Cooper, M.D.—Director, The Aerobics Institute, Dallas, Texas

Steven Corson, M.D.—Director, Philadelphia Fertility Institute; Clinical Professor of Obstetrics and Gynecology, University of Pennsylvania School of Medicine, Philadelphia, PA

David Costil, Ph.D.—Director, Human Performance Laboratory, Ball State University, Muncie, IN

James Cusumano, Ph.D.—Chairman, Catalytica, Inc., Palo Alto, CA

Kenneth Davis, M.D.—Chairman, Department of Psychiatry, Mt. Sinai School of Medicine, New York, NY

Edward Dietrich, M.D.—Medical Director/Chairman of Cardiovascular Surgery, Arizona Heart Institute, Phoenix, AZ

Larry Dossey, M.D.—Author, *Meaning and Medicine; Recovering the Soul; Beyond Illness; Space, Time and Medicine;* Santa Fe, NM

David Eddy, M.D., Ph.D.—Professor of Health Policy and Management, Duke University School of Medicine, Durham, NC

Charles Edwards, M.D.—President, Scripps Clinics and Hospital, La Jolla, CA; former Commissioner, Food and Drug Administration

Alain Enthoven, Ph.D.—Professor of Business, Graduate School of Business, Stanford University, Stanford, CA

William Evans, Ph.D.—Chief, Human Physiology Laboratory, The USDA Human Nutrition Research Center on Aging, Tufts University, Boston, MA

Margaret Fischl, M.D.—Chairman, AIDS Clinical Trials Group, National Institutes of Health; Professor of Medicine, University of Miami School of Medicine, Miami, FL

Theodore Friedmann, M.D.—Professor of Medicine, Division of Molecular Genetics, University of California, San Diego School of Medicine, San Diego, CA

Robert Glickman, M.D.—Physician-in-Chief, Beth Israel Hospital; Professor of Medicine, Harvard Medical School, Boston, MA

Paul Goldhaber, D.M.D.—Dean Emeritus, Harvard School of Dental Medicine, Boston, MA

Robert Good, M.D., Ph.D.—Physician-in-Chief, All Children's Hospital, Professor of Pediatrics, University of South Florida School of Medicine, St. Petersburg, FL

Alain Grisel, Ph.D.—President, Microsens, Neuchâtel, Switzerland

Scott Grundy, M.D., Ph.D.—Director, Institute for Human Nutrition, Professor of Medicine and Biochemistry, University of Texas, Southwestern Medical School at Dallas, Dallas, TX

Leroy Hood, M.D., Ph.D.—Chairman, Department of Molecular Biotechnology, University of Washington School of Medicine, Seattle, WA

William Hrushesky, M.D.—Professor of Medicine and Immunobiology, Albany Medical College, Albany, NY

Axel Kahn, M.D.—Institut Cochin de Genetique Moleculaire, Paris, France

Norman Kaplan, M.D.—Professor of Medicine, Division of Hypertension, University of Texas Southwestern Medical Center at Dallas, Dallas, TX

Edwin Kilbourne, M.D.—Chairman, Department of Microbiology, Mt. Sinai School of Medicine, New York, NY

Donald Klein, M.D.—New York State Psychiatric Institute; Professor of Psychiatry, Columbia University School of Medicine, New York, NY

Alfred Knudsen, M.D., Ph.D.—Senior Member, Fox Chase Cancer Center, Philadelphia, PA; Adjunct Professor, Pediatrics and Human Genetics, University of Pennsylvania School of Medicine, Philadelphia, PA

Mark Lappin, Esq.—Partner, Lahive and Cockfield, Attorneys at Law, Boston, MA

M. Rigdon Lentz, M.D.—Chairman, Innatus Foundation for Cancer Research, Indio, CA

Richard Lerner, M.D.—Director, Scripps Clinic and Hospitals Research Foundation, La Jolla, CA

Robert Lindsay, M.D., Ph.D.—Director, Bone Research Unit and Chief of Medicine, Helen Hayes Hospital, West Haverstraw, NY; Professor of Medicine, Columbia University School of Medicine, New York, NY

Susan Love, M.D.—Director, Faulkner Breast Center, Boston, MA; Professor of Surgery, Dana Farber Hospital, Harvard Medical School, Boston, MA            .

George Lundberg, M.D.—President 1989–1990, American Society of Clinical Pathology; Vice-President for Scientific Affairs, American Medical Association; Editor-in-Chief, *Journal of the American Medical Association*, Chicago, IL

Ryan Mathews—Editor-in-Chief, *Progressive Grocer*, Gorman Publications, Detroit, MI

John McAfee, M.D.—Professor of Nuclear Medicine, George Washington University School of Medicine, Washington, DC

Stephen McNamara, Esq.—Partner, Hyman Phelps and McNamara, Attorneys at Law, Washington, DC

Elliot Middleton, M.D.—Professor of Medicine and Allergy, State University of New York at Buffalo School of Medicine, Buffalo, NY

Martin Moore-Ede, M.D., Ph.D.—Director, Institute for Circadian Physiology, Boston, MA

Elizabeth Nabel, M.D.—Associate Professor, Division of Medicine and Cardiology, University of Michigan Medical School, Ann Arbor, MI

Ernest Noble, Ph.D., M.D.—Pike Professor of Alcohol Studies and Director, Alcohol Research Unit, UCLA Medical School, Los Angeles, CA

Robert Oldham, M.D.—Director, Biological Therapy Institute, Franklin, TN

Norman Orentreich, M.D.—Director, Orentreich Foundation for the Advancement of Science; Professor of Dermatology, New York University School of Medicine, New York, NY

Gerald Pohost, M.D.—Director, Cardiac Imaging Center, University of Alabama School of Medicine, Birmingham, AL

William Regelson, M.D.—Professor of Medicine, Medical College of Virginia, Richmond, VA

Isadore Rosenfeld, M.D.—Professor of Medicine, Division of Cardiology, New York Hospital–Cornell Medical Center, New York, NY

Mace Rothenberg, M.D.—Director of Alternative Therapies, National Cancer Institute, Bethesda, MD

David Sachs, M.D.—Director, Transplantation Biology Research Center, Massachusetts General Hospital; Paul S. Russell/Warner Lambert Professor of Surgery, Harvard Medical School, Boston, MA

Daniel Schneck, Ph.D.—Professor, Engineering, Science and Mechanics, Virginia Polytechnic Institute, Blacksburg, VA

Paul Segall, Ph.D.—Chairman, BioTime Inc., Berkeley, CA

William Silen, M.D.—Surgeon-in-Chief, Beth Israel Hospital; Professor of Surgery, Harvard Medical School, Boston, MA

Clement Sledge, M.D.—Chairman, Department of Orthopedics, Brigham and Women's Hospital; Professor of Orthopedics, Harvard Medical School, Boston, MA

Redmond Smith, M.D.—Editor, *British Journal of Ophthalmology*, London, UK

Solomon Snyder, M.D., Ph.D.—Chairman, Department of Neurosciences, Johns Hopkins University School of Medicine, Baltimore, MD

M. Therese Southgate, M.D.—Cover Editor, *Journal of the American Medical Association;* Professor of Medical Ethics, Northwestern University Medical School, Chicago, IL

Robert Swanson—Chairman, Genentech, Inc., South San Francisco, CA

Patrick Walsh, M.D.—Chairman, Department of Urology, Professor of Urology, Johns Hopkins University School of Medicine, Baltimore, MD

Nancy Wexler, Ph.D.—New York State Psychiatric Institute, Columbia University, New York, NY; President, Hereditary Disease Foundation, Los Angeles, CA

Joseph Williams—Former Chairman and CEO, Warner Lambert Co., Morris Plains, NJ

Morris Ziff, M.D., Ph.D.—Professor Emeritus of Medicine and Rheumatology, University of Texas Southwestern Medical School at Dallas, Dallas, TX

Adrian Zorgniotti, M.D.—Professor of Urology, New York University School of Medicine, New York, NY

# Introduction: An Intimate Technology

THE STRIKING PARADOX ABOUT MEDICINE'S FUTURE IS THAT TECH-
nology—the cold surface of scientific progress that most of us fear
as impersonal—will, in fact, eventually allow us to literally *see* our
biological uniqueness. Tools more miraculous than most of us can
now imagine will force upon practitioners a view of their patients
that cannot be generalized into quick labels or facile categories.
The practice of medicine will be charged with an unprecedented
excitement when doctors are actually able to look inside every one
of our trillions of cells and detect any abnormalities at the most
basic molecular level, long before we experience symptoms. The
prevention of disease will thus become the most important component of medical practice. And eventually, our ability to prevent
will be enhanced by our ability to predict. Most of the diseases we
now fear are going to become so rare as to be curiosities, in fact
newsworthy when they occur.

"Prediction" is really another way of saying "early detection"—
so early that we can alter *predisease* metabolic abnormalities at the
molecular level. If one is unluckily born with a predisposition for
coronary heart disease we will discover it early enough to take steps

to prevent it before it occurs. The same opportunity would be true of a susceptibility to cancer or any other ailment.

At birth, or in some cases even before birth, everyone will have a fully automated diagnostic biochemical profile performed on the smallest imaginable biopsy specimen—a fragment of one cell. This profile will predict a patient's predisposition to specific diseases, and the results will become part of our permanent medical record. The predictions will be so accurate that they will provide information about not only what disease one is most likely to get later in life but what cellular abnormality is likely to make us most vulnerable. Physicians will then, at the appropriate time, reach into their future version of the doctor's bag and administer the warranted remedial therapy.

The use of this predictive ability, especially when combined with the new preventive methodology, will be a godsend to patients and physicians. The anxiety of the unknown will be eliminated, along with the disease. Young people growing up will no longer fear such conditions as hereditary cancer or heart disease. The doctor of today has no legitimate prognosticating implements and can only use family history as a guide, a sometimes helpful but relatively crude means of estimating future risk. The physician of the future will be a medical astrologer of sorts, but the horoscope-like reading that she or he gives to patients will be based on the best that science has to offer.

What is this technology that is going to fuel these sweeping transitions? When the American biologist James Watson and British physicist Francis Crick figured out the structure of DNA in 1953, the entire approach to biology and genetics was changed. No longer was science involved with naming and classifying animals and plants and breeding fruit flies in the laboratory; now it was studying what happens inside cells at the most basic level. The sciences of molecular biology and molecular genetics were born. Although it was known at the time to be a monumental breakthrough (for which Watson and Crick were awarded the Nobel Prize in medicine in 1962), like most great discoveries it inspired more questions than it answered.

Over the following four decades, scientists around the world have been working at solving the huge jigsaw puzzle uncovered by Watson and Crick. It is now well established that DNA is the seat of all the genes in every cell in the body, and therefore to a large extent controls every one of our characteristics. This includes physical traits such as eye color and height; biochemical traits such as how we metabolize fat and cholesterol and how well our immune systems function; talent and ability such as how well we remember things, paint, or play tennis; and even many personality characteristics such as whether we are extroverted or introverted.

Intensive study by scientists involved in the $3 billion Human Genome Project is revealing the exact location on the DNA molecule of each of the 100,000 genes, and determining precisely which genes do what. But this knowledge supplies only one crucial piece of the puzzle. In order for physicians to be able to manipulate what the genes have preordained, to actually change a predisposition for disease, it is first necessary to understand exactly how the genes interact to orchestrate the incredibly complex cascade of biochemical and electronic messages and controls that constitute cellular metabolism.

Using the tools that have been developed in molecular genetics, molecular biology and biotechnology, scientists are making astounding progress toward understanding the genetic and molecular workings of the cell, and thereby the underpinnings of disease at the most basic and earliest level (in many cases even before it begins). Just as the Hubble Telescope is observing the planets, these molecular spies are looking inside the cell and discovering an extraordinary amount about exactly how both normal and abnormal cells function. The more that is learned about how cells function, the more we can do to keep normal cells from becoming abnormal and to alter the function of abnormal cells to make them normal. The fact that this research has taken so many brilliant researchers so long is testimony to the complexity of the human machinery. Of course, the work is nowhere near completion. The biochemical journey that lies ahead is a long one, but a critical mass of knowledge has already been accumulated. Not only will future progress come much faster but we are now at the point when we can begin applying this wisdom to clinical treatments.

Many future breakthroughs are in fact already in the early stages of development and we can now sketch the dramatic scenarios of change that will constitute the major trends of the years ahead. We will see our concept of reproduction and parenthood dramatically changed by genetic engineering, molecular diagnostics and in vitro fertilization. By the year 2020 it will be possible to have a child—that is, go from conception to birth—entirely outside the human body, as the result of the perfection of an artificial placenta.

Furthermore, we will be able to produce newborns who are disease-free and genetically programmed for whatever talents, abilities and level of intelligence we choose.

The new technology is going to provide us with ultimate control of our bodies after birth. Our knowledge of a person's genetic profile will transform the science of organ transplants by enabling us to ensure immunological compatibility between donor and recipient. Replacing damaged or diseased body parts will become a minor operation, with almost no risk factor involved. This will be taken even one step further beginning only a decade after the millennium when the use of artificial organs enables us to remake the human mechanism in a fashion heretofore envisioned only in science fiction.

The tremendous advances in genetics, molecular biology and neuropharmacology will also be applied to the brain, giving us the know-how to end all forms of addiction, from smoking and overeating to narcotics, and to safely and effectively manipulate our emotions.

As for our lives at home, beginning in about ten years, an astonishing array of new medical equipment will be as standard as televisions or microwaves are now. We will soon have the capability of performing certain routine blood tests on ourselves without drawing blood, and by 2020 technological advances will allow us to screen ourselves for a broad spectrum of early cellular abnormalities while we take our morning shower.

Finally, *what* we do to diagnose, treat and prevent disease will be perfected by knowing exactly *when* to do it. As chronobiologists zero in on how our biological clocks cause metabolic variations, we will be able to identify vulnerability to a disease at the earliest possible moment and intervene to stop the pathology.

When are all these miracles going to occur? Dare we give dates to our predictions? Yes. Based on research in science and medicine that is currently under way, we can confidently assemble an extensive timeline running year by year from 1992 to 2030: a chronicle of cures we can expect, and when we can expect them for every major illness and minor ailment, as well as a list of problems we can prevent and therefore eliminate from our list of things to worry about.

The ethical questions inherent in all the exciting and good news are already being acknowledged and addressed with caution by the scientific community, and I will discuss these moral dilemmas in the chapters that follow and, finally, in the summary epilogue. But, ultimately, nourished and sustained by the molecular revolutions, the medicine of the future will work with the body rather than against it, bringing to health care a solution that is both technologically brilliant and consummately humane.

# PART

## I

# TRENDS

# 1

# The Ultimate Separation of Sex and Reproduction

FOLK WISDOM TELLS US THAT THE MORE THINGS CHANGE, THE more they remain the same. And until very recently there didn't seem to be a reason to challenge an adage that so succinctly sums up humankind's way of clinging to comfortable habits and familiar behaviors in the face of social disruptions. But if one of our most basic givens about family life were one day so radically challenged that nothing in human relations could ever be the same again, we would have to alter that adage and say instead: the more things change, the more we are changed forever.

That day is not all that far in the future. It will arrive, precipitously, on the heels of a technology that will challenge the simplest, everyday assumptions about how we have babies. We believe that day will come by the year 1998.

It has been difficult enough educating our relatively puritanical society about sex and reproduction as it has existed for hundreds of millions of years. And most of that education has been crammed into the past forty years. By the time the possibilities of psychologically enhanced sex and medically assisted procreation came along, it seemed we had more to think about than we could comfortably handle.

But because we've been on such an accelerated learning curve, our ability to adapt to change has evolved. The majority of us are now willing to condone practicing whatever sexual behaviors consenting adults find appropriate, as long as they keep it indoors and away from children. So we will quickly adapt as well to the changes in how babies are made.

Because of these changes, we are going to have to redefine our notions of what motherhood, fatherhood and pregnancy are. Some women will become biological mothers but won't get pregnant, hiring a birth mother instead. Other women will choose to become pregnant later in life, after their careers and even after menopause, either by carrying their own embryo conceived years earlier or by buying eggs from another woman. Some women will become pregnant without meeting the father. Men will become biological fathers without meeting the mother. Some babies will be born without anyone becoming pregnant at all! And there are other permutations as well.

Undoubtedly, many of us will initially find these ideas too abhorrent, too foreign to the basic human way of life. What right do science and medicine have to intrude upon this most natural of life processes and make it so unnatural? This sort of ethical question is going to come up again and again in the future of health care, and not just in the area of reproduction. How we answer it will ultimately depend upon circumstances.

Although most advances in the manipulation of the reproductive process have come about through high-tech procedures developed in the past fifteen years, this field of medicine actually began long ago when, in 1799, a British physician named John Hunter performed the first successful artificial insemination. This innovative doctor didn't need technology to achieve results, just a bit of clear thinking. He recommended to a patient who had a deformed penis that he put his semen into a syringelike device and push it into his wife's vagina. Miraculously, it was successful and a healthy baby was delivered. Artificial insemination was introduced in the United States shortly thereafter. The procedures have, of course, been refined since then but the basic concept remains the same: the assisted insertion of sperm into the reproductive tract of the female, either the vagina or cervix or directly into the uterus.

The use of sperm from a donor other than the husband or regular sexual partner of the woman is an innovation that stems from John Hunter's original idea but not, as you might imagine, a modern one. Surprisingly, this variant technique was performed for the first time at Jefferson Hospital in Philadelphia in 1882. It was quite a leap from there to 1988 and the celebrated case of Mary Beth Whitehead and Baby M., in which a husband's sperm was used to inseminate a donor woman. But now things are moving much more quickly.

The prospects for infertile couples increased enormously with the development of techniques for fertilization outside the body known as *in vitro fertilization,* or IVF. This was successfully used in 1978 by British physicians Robert Edwards and Patrick Steptoe and culminated in the arrival of Louise Brown, the world's first test-tube baby.

As with both types of artificial insemination, this technology was introduced to help couples who couldn't conceive by natural means. The most common reason for in vitro fertilization is blocked oviducts (fallopian tubes) in the woman. When this condition exists, even if egg and sperm are healthy and eager to meet, they find their path blocked. To circumvent this, eggs are removed from the woman, fertilized in a glass dish in the laboratory by the husband's sperm, and the resultant embryo is then implanted in the wife's uterus and allowed to develop.

After some initial success, in vitro fertility clinics sprang up all over the world and, although expensive (about six to eight thousand dollars) and often not covered by medical insurance, drew many couples to them. The uses of IVF have been extended beyond women with blocked oviducts to those with endometriosis, those with antibodies against sperm and those couples who have unexplained infertility.

In vitro fertility is being used to solve problems of male infertility as well. It is now known that as much as 30 to 40 percent of infertility is due to the male. The technique has application to the same males who can be helped by artificial insemination, that is, those who are subfertile, but not completely infertile.

The evolution of in vitro fertilization in just a little more than a decade has been truly amazing, opening avenues to more than twenty thousand couples who otherwise would have been unable to conceive. Considering the size of the total population, twenty thousand is still a relatively small number. Only about one in six couples is infertile and not all of them need the high technology of in vitro fertilization to solve their problems.

But as we head into the twenty-first century and beyond, there is going to be a fundamental and startling change in the use of this technology: the use of in vitro fertilization by people who are perfectly capable of conceiving by natural means. IVF will become a routine method of conceiving children and, because of its widespread use and the consequent competition among suppliers, the costs of some of the more basic procedures will go down, bringing this alternative within the reach of many more people.

The expansion of reproductive choices will spawn career opportunities in preembryo, genetic testing labs, and in egg and sperm banks. There will be entrepreneurial egg and sperm speculators, jobs for surrogates and a whole range of ancillary supporting occupations, as well as increased demand for reproductive biologists and reproductive consultants.

In order to better appreciate what is coming, it will help to follow the progression of events from just a few years in the future, where things won't seem too unfamiliar, all the way to 2020 and beyond, where things are going to look decidedly different.

It is late August 1998 and a young married couple, in their early thirties and perfectly healthy, feel the time has come to have their first child. On their own they make no effort at achieving pregnancy; instead they visit an obstetrician with a list of their needs and preferences. First: they've decided on the sex of their child—they want a boy—and this choice can be 100 percent guaranteed. Second: the woman is a busy accountant and would like to time her pregnancy so that delivery doesn't come during tax season. The remaining items on their list cover the more familiar concerns regarding health and well-being.

To accommodate their wishes they will have to spend about five thousand dollars and put up with some minor inconvenience at the start. Their physician will be happy to manage the prenatal care once pregnancy ensues, but there are prepregnancy steps that will have to be overseen at a reproductive choice center.

At the center, the couple meet with a counselor who describes himself as a trained reproductive biologist. The counselor takes them into a softly lit, well-appointed room with large comfortable chairs, a wide television screen and a variety of video equipment and shows them a fifteen-minute film that explains the three basic steps they will have to undergo: in vitro fertilization, preembryo testing, and finally implantation into the uterus.

In the past, it was possible to determine the sex of the baby only after pregnancy had already occurred—either through amniocentesis or a newer technique called chorionic villus sampling. Amniocentesis is done at about sixteen to eighteen weeks of pregnancy by inserting a large needle into the amniotic sac in which the fetus is developing, culturing the cells in the laboratory and then examining them under a microscope. Not only can chromosome abnormalities such as Down's syndrome be detected, but also the sex of the baby. Chorionic villus sampling is done earlier—at about eight weeks—and involves snipping a piece of the placenta and looking for the same things.

Now though, the film explains, it is possible to determine the baby's sex before pregnancy, which totally circumvents the question of whether or not to perform an abortion for sex selection. The egg will be fertilized outside the body and tested for sexual identity before being implanted in the uterus.

Before in vitro fertilization can occur, however, several eggs must be collected from the prospective mother's ovaries, not only to guarantee that there will be some mature eggs to fertilize but, since they are only interested in "male-producing" eggs, so that several can be fertilized to assure that.

The woman will have to take ovulation-inducing drugs such as Pergonal and Luprolide which cause many eggs to develop simultaneously in one menstrual cycle. While she is taking the drugs, her estrogen levels (which influence egg maturation) will be watched and she will be closely monitored with ultrasonic examination to identify the developing follicles. At the appropriate development time, she will be given an injection of a hormone called human chorionic gonadotropin or hCG to induce final maturation. About thirty-six hours later, under local anesthesia, the eggs will be retrieved from the ovary by means of a computer-guided needle inserted through the vagina. Although this procedure is relatively simple and only moderately noninvasive there is always a very slight danger of the needle causing some residual bleeding or infection.

The mature eggs will be placed in organ culture dishes which contain a special insemination medium, while the immature eggs are placed in an incubator to mature further. The woman's husband then produces a fresh sample of semen from which the most motile sperm are identified. These are placed in the organ culture dish with the mature eggs and treated with a mild enzyme to dissolve the outer membrane of the egg, or the membrane is penetrated with a microscopic drill or a laser. Each of these procedures makes it easier for fertilization to occur.

After it has been determined microscopically that fertilization has occurred, the fertilized eggs are put into an incubator while the procedure is repeated with the now more-ripened eggs that have been incubating. These are added to the other fertilized eggs until they have all divided three times, so that they are now each a clump of eight cells. These clumps of cells are called preembryos, a totally new term that arose from in vitro fertilization technology. Technically, a true embryo doesn't begin until implantation in the uterus, so preembryos are one step before that.

The next step will be to remove one of the cells from each clump of eight and subject them to an automated biochemical and morphological analysis that will predict viability of the preembryo. After it has been determined that a preembryo's cell is "healthy," laboratory technicians then subject that same cell to a series of procedures that extract all the DNA. This DNA will then be amplified billions of times by a sequence of enzymatic steps called the polymerase chain reaction. This creates enough DNA to react with a molecular probe that will identify whether the Y chromosome (denoting a male) is present. If it is absent, the preembryo is a female.

The desired "male" preembryo will now be transferred to a culture dish where it will remain for forty-eight hours, growing in a medium that contains cells from the lining of the fallopian tube. This step significantly increases its chances for a successful implantation when it is inserted into the uterus by means of a long needle and a syringe. Other "backup" preembryos are kept in the culture medium in case the implantation doesn't take. The remainder of the pregnancy will proceed as if it had occurred by natural means, and nine months later a baby boy will be delivered. Since the fertilization is done in vitro, it will be possible to take ovulation-inducing drugs during any cycle, so that it can coincide with the month the couple want their baby to be born.

After they have viewed the instructional film, the reproductive biologist makes certain that the couple understands that the unused preembryos will be discarded, and needs to determine that they have no objection to that. When they assure him that they do not, they are advised to come back the following day and meet with the physician who will be directing their program. At that appointment, it is suggested that the woman begin taking the ovulation-inducing and follicle-maturing drugs the following month. Although this woman will be pregnant during tax season, she won't be near enough to term for it to interfere with her work.

In 1998, sex selection and the timing of pregnancy won't be the only reasons for choosing in vitro fertilization. As this couple leaves the reproductive choice center, they notice two other couples.

The first man and woman will undergo almost the same procedure as the previous couple, except that they are not interested in the sex of their baby, only its health. The woman has had two previous pregnancies end unhappily. The first one nine years ago had been disastrous. Their baby had been born with the deadly neurological malady Tay-Sachs disease and had lived a vegetative existence for three years until it mercifully died. The couple was so devastated that they waited six years until attempting pregnancy again. This time, chorionic villus sampling at eight weeks revealed that this fetus also had Tay-Sachs disease, and the pregnancy was terminated.

Although aborting the pregnancy hadn't been nearly as traumatic as their first experience, the couple is understandably reluctant to attempt pregnancy again. The physician at the center assures them, however, that this time they won't have to endure such painful disappointment.

They will follow essentially the same procedure as for sex selection except that the preembryos will be tested for the presence of Tay-Sachs disease, rather than examined for sexual identity (that could be done as well, but this couple actually prefers not to know). As with other recessive conditions such as cystic fibrosis, both parents must be carriers and pass that gene on to their children for them to be afflicted—only a one-in-four chance with each pregnancy—so this couple has been unlucky. But since the drugs the woman will take during a menstrual cycle will cause more than one of her eggs to ripen, there will be several chances to produce a preembryo that is free of the Tay-Sachs gene. It is almost mathematically incomprehensible that at least one healthy, Tay-Sachs-disease-free preembryo won't be created, and even if it did happen, all of the preembryos could be discarded and the procedure repeated a few months later.

Once the eggs have been collected and fertilized with her husband's sperm, they will be tested in much the same way as for sex selection, except that this will involve looking for a specific gene, rather than a whole chromosome as is done for sex selection. All this entails, though, is an additional step. After the DNA is extracted from one of the viable preembryo cells, it is subjected to specific enzymes that will cut the DNA and isolate the region that is known to harbor the Tay-Sachs gene. This segment will then be treated as before—amplified with the polymerase chain reaction to produce enough of the material to test—and then reacted with a molecular probe that will detect the presence or absence of the Tay-Sachs gene.

The procedure, as predicted, is completely successful. More than one viable, Tay-Sachs-free preembryo is identified and one is inserted into the woman's uterus. She is sent back to her obstetrician for prenatal care, with blessed peace of mind, knowing that in nine months she is going to deliver a healthy baby.

Although genetic testing of this sort will still be in its early stages in 1998, it will be possible to detect a variety of conditions such as cystic fibrosis, Down's syndrome, sickle cell disease, Huntington's disease and other so-called one-gene conditions. These "simply inherited" diseases have an uncomplicated inheritance pattern. (All "simply inherited" diseases, dominant or recessive, are called "one-gene" diseases.) For dominant conditions such as Huntington's disease, the presence of only one copy of the gene from either parent indicates the eventual appearance of the disease (although Huntington's disease doesn't manifest itself until much later in life—symptoms usually begin in the fifth or sixth decade—its presence is determined at the moment of conception). For recessive conditions, such as Tay-Sachs disease or cystic fibrosis, the fertilized egg must carry two copies of the gene for the disease to occur. With one copy, the offspring would only be a carrier. DNA testing on preembryos will be able to determine either of these occurrences.

The other couple in the waiting room has yet another reason for choosing in vitro fertilization. The woman, thirty-five years old, has just begun her own business and knows that she will have to devote the next ten years or so to nurturing it. Her company will be her only child until she is at least forty-five years old. She wants to have a baby one day but knows that she won't be ready until she reaches a day when safe conception is questionable.

In vitro fertilization offers a solution to this couple's dilemma. But now, instead of the preembryo being immediately implanted in the woman's uterus, it will be carefully identified and frozen until she is ready to become pregnant and have her baby ten or more years down the line. Then the cryopreserved preembryo will be thawed, cultured in oviduct cells for a couple of days to aid in implantation, and inserted into her uterus. The most viable preembryos will have been chosen, and in 1998 newly invented techniques for optimum freezing and eventual thawing will keep the preembryo healthy. By 2008 or later, when this woman is ready to become pregnant, much more will be known about the hormonal and immunological factors, both maternal and fetal, that govern successful implantation in the uterus than was known years earlier. While the preembryo is being prepared for implantation, the mother will be made ready with implantation-enhancing hormones.

Time will be on this couple's side in other ways. If they desire, they can select the sex of their child ten years in advance. And by the time the preembryo is thawed for implantation it will be possible to test for myriad genetic problems. Since several potentially viable preembryos will have been frozen, they will each be subjected to genetic analyses before implantation. A preembryo that might have seemed perfectly healthy in 1998 may not any longer fall into that category in 2008. The child who is chosen for birth in 2008 will be more genetically fit than one born ten years earlier.

By 1998 it will be possible for a woman either to have her own eggs collected and fertilized by her partner's sperm or to buy an egg from an anonymous donor, in which case her baby won't carry her genes at all, but only those of her partner and the donor.

The availability of egg donation creates still other alternatives. For years it has been possible to successfully cryopreserve sperm and have them retain their ability to fertilize eggs when thawed. Their capacity is somewhat diminished as compared with fresh sperm, but just as progress will be made in understanding optimum conditions for preserving the viability of frozen preembryos, so will it be made with sperm. By 1998, there will be little difference between the fertilizing capabilities of fresh and frozen sperm.

Although by 1998 the technology for freezing eggs won't be fully developed, using frozen sperm and fresh eggs from donors will allow for many reproductive combinations. Single women will be able to have their own eggs collected and fertilized with anonymously donated frozen sperm they have chosen. There are already several facilities where sperm can be procured, and there will be many more in 1998. Since genetic testing will still be in its early stages, what a woman buying this sperm will be able to tell about her purchase will be limited to basic issues of health and disease, but the facility where the sperm is bought will have information about the donor on file, such as height, weight, eye and hair color, and level of education. Later, the preembryo will be tested as further insurance against a genetic problem.

As I sit back and imagine this scenario as a way of testing my own deepest feelings about this brave new world of alternate families, I think of what my response might be to a child of mine choosing this method of parenthood. And then I realize that the issue is already familiar. It was not so long ago that our parents were taken aback by the whole notion of scheduled births, yet now it is perfectly common for a woman to plan to have her child by cesarean section to work around the all-important board meeting, or family vacation, or whatever scheduling problem she is facing. For that matter, it wasn't many years ago that society doubted the competence of those who chose to be single parents. But single parenting is now recognized as one of the realities of our world. When I think of it this way, I realize that often the biggest problems have to do with the rapidity of change. The changes in our reproductive options will provoke ethical questions that each of us must resolve personally. As we become better informed, perhaps the shiver of apprehension about the future will give way to the calm of reasoned discussion and, for many, acceptance.

Whatever one's point of view, the fact is that surrogate parenting will be reasonably well established by 1998. A single male who wants to have a child can have his sperm utilized to fertilize an anonymously donated egg and the preembryo can then be tested and either frozen for later implantation or implanted in a uterus right away. But the carrier of the fetus will not be the egg donor. That was what caused so much difficulty in the Mary Beth Whitehead case. Now a surrogate parent will be a third party, who doesn't donate either egg or sperm, whose uterus is "rented" for nine months. After delivery, the baby will belong to whoever bought the egg and rented the uterus.

Both egg donation and surrogate carriers will be occupations in their incipient stages of development in 1998, still not fully organized but utilized frequently. As we journey further into the future, to 2010, we find that not only has this aspect of reproductive control been advanced but several new options have come along.

In 1998, sexual identity and the presence of simply inherited one-gene diseases, such as Tay Sachs disease, will be the only analyses that will be available in reproductive clinics. By 2010, however, it will be possible to test preembryos not only for the guaranteed presence of a disease, but even for the *susceptibility* to a disease sometime after birth. This will include many relatively common diseases—cardiovascular disease, cancer, Alzheimer's disease, diabetes, manic depression, and even some rather minor conditions such as allergies.

The development of commercial tests for these disorders will parallel progression of the Human Genome Project. The work of the project is scheduled for completion by 2005. Susceptibility to an ailment depends on the presence or absence of a whole set of genes whose impact is additive. We're no longer talking about just one gene. To put the difficulty of such an undertaking in perspective, consider the fact that even in a mouse a seemingly simple trait such as hair and skin color requires the interaction of more than one hundred forty-seven genes as determinants. The number of genes that control similar traits in humans is almost certainly greater and those that control disease susceptibility much greater still.

Pursuing their goal inexorably, the scientists in the Human Genome Project will eventually identify the molecular addresses of every disease-related gene, and once that's done there will be commercially available tests for each of them. We're calling for that to happen by 2010, and laboratories that specialize in preembryo testing will then become an integral part of reproductive centers.

Because prospective parents who have IVF-created preembryos tested will be given much more information in 2010 than in 1998, they will face more difficult choices. Discarding a clump of cells that carries a gene for muscular dystrophy doesn't involve much soul-searching, but doing away with a preembryo that carries a susceptibility for a relatively benign condition such as asthma (or even cardiovascular disease, which requires exposure to environmental factors before the set of predisposing genes will ever be expressed) will involve some difficult decisions.

Our preconceived notions about what our babies should be are certain to change as science progresses. As Dr. Arthur Caplan, director of the Center for Biomedical Ethics at the University of Minnesota School of Medicine, told me, "The expectation as to what constitutes a malady will go up in direct proportion to our ability to screen out and eliminate these conditions." Many of us will come to expect, almost demand, a perfect preembryo.

So far there's been no breakthrough in egg-freezing technology, in humans or animals, and this is either because eggs are older than sperm (women are born with their full complement of eggs whereas men continue to produce sperm most of their lives) or because of inherent properties of eggs that resist freezing. But several researchers in the field, including Dr. Aldo Campana of the department of obstetrics and gynecology of the University of Geneva, are confident it will be accomplished by 2010. When I met with Dr. Campana in his office in Switzerland in the fall of 1990 he told me of a report of a successful egg freezing, thawing and subsequent pregnancy in China. Although it had not yet been duplicated, Dr. Campana was sanguine about the chances of its happening.

The ability to freeze and bank eggs will open the door to several new reproductive choices, especially when combined with the expanded genetic testing that will be available. Fresh egg donation, in which it is more difficult for the donor to remain anonymous and which requires almost immediate decisions by those procuring the donated egg, will be replaced by frozen egg banking by 2010. This will allow for not only more choices about which egg to obtain but, since they will be frozen, more control over when the purchase will be made.

It will be possible to perform the same genetic analyses on frozen eggs and sperm in 2010 as on preembryos. Fortunately, nature has provided a convenient way for this to be done even on a fragile egg. During maturation, an egg produces and discards a small, discrete substance called a polar body, which contains the full complement of genetic material found in the mature egg DNA. Rather than disturb the egg and risk damaging it, genetic testing will be performed on the polar body, which will yield the same information.

The eggs and sperm of anonymous donors will be genetically

tested and, if found to be free of any disease-related genes and disease-susceptibility-related genes, will be catalogued and stored along with their physical and social characteristics. Since these donors will be a valuable resource for the egg and sperm banks, they will be regularly paid to donate.

Those who will be producing their babies from donated sperm and eggs will go to a facility directly related to the reproductive center—an "egg adoption clinic" or "sperm adoption clinic," depending on which they want to "adopt." They will purchase an already guaranteed genetically disease-free egg or sperm that has been donated by someone with characteristics they desire. This will then be combined in vitro with their corresponding egg or sperm and fertilization will take place. Since genes from the egg and sperm combine at random, and therefore the composition of the fertilized egg can't be accurately predicted, the resultant preembryo will still need to be subjected to genetic analysis, but it will give adopters of egg and sperm much more control over the starting material than will be available pre-2010.

Many of the pregnancies that begin this way will require the participation of a third party to carry the baby to term. Older women who buy eggs or who had their preembryos frozen several years earlier will very likely use a third party rather than carry the baby themselves, even though as early as 1991 it was possible for a fifty-two-year-old woman to successfully carry a baby to term. By 2010, being a surrogate carrier will be a well-defined career option for many women.

The requirements for the job of surrogate will be relative youth (being under forty), enjoying pregnancy and being in exceptionally good health. Additional requirements will include being a non-smoker, agreeing not to drink at all while pregnant, having normal blood pressure, being in good athletic condition and passing a psychological stress test. Since the surrogate will not contribute genes, race won't be a factor. Surrogates will be extremely well paid and will not meet the prospective parent or parents at all. The choice of the surrogate will be made at random from those available through the surrogate agency, and all negotiations with the parents will be handled by attorneys who represent the agency and who specialize in surrogacy law.

The surrogates will live under controlled conditions while they are pregnant, in a "surrogacy spa," a facility funded out of fees paid by the prospective parents. It will combine a fully equipped obstetric clinic and hospital with a luxury resort. The surrogate will eat specially prepared diets, and reside in a completely stress-free environment, with all of her needs met. There will be access to all forms of exercise, entertainment and intellectual stimulation. The surrogates will be examined regularly by highly trained physicians-in-residence who will give them advanced prenatal care. It will involve not only the standard prenatal care of today—monitoring weight gain and blood pressure and administering prenatal vitamins—but a more positive form of care, in which each surrogate will take substances to provide an optimal growth environment for the fetus.

Delivery of the baby will be at the surrogacy spa, and immediately thereafter the baby will be taken to the home of its legal parents, where there will be an obstetric nurse to monitor the baby for the first few days. In order to make the transition smooth, the legal mother and the surrogate will take hormonal substances that will have opposite effects on their emotional attachment to the child.

In the early days of surrogacy, in the 1990s, it was discovered that even if the gestational carrier made no genetic contribution to the baby, she would still experience a psychological bonding with the child and not want to relinquish it. At that time it was felt that this would present a genuine impediment to the widespread use of surrogates.

However, it has also been discovered that the bonding process was mediated by a simple, small hormone, a peptide called oxytocin. For many years it was known that oxytocin plays a crucial role in uterine contractions during labor and stimulates the flow of milk in breast-feeding mothers, but it wasn't until the early 1990s that it was found to play a role in bonding.

By 2010, this role will have been clearly elucidated. Since oxytocin has a wide range of functions, synthetic analogues will be developed to specifically modulate bonding without affecting the other actions of oxytocin. Beginning a month before the surrogate gives birth to her child, the genetic mother will take this oxytocinlike substance to stimulate feelings of bonding with her soon-to-arrive baby. She will also have been taking hormones to induce lactation, so the oxytocin will help begin the flow of breast milk with which she will feed her baby.

Meanwhile, all during her pregnancy the surrogate will have been taking drugs to inhibit the specific bonding effect of oxytocin, without impeding the uterine contractions she will need during delivery. The effects of this oxytocin-blocker will be quickly reversible once discontinued and will not prevent the surrogate from being a loving mother herself.

Ten years further out, by 2020, genetic testing will no longer be limited to the detection of disease-related susceptibilities. Now it will be applied to human abilities, and physical and personality traits as well. This is when the stakes get higher.

Although environment plays a role in the development of abilities and personality characteristics similar to the one it plays in the expression of diseases for which a susceptibility has been inherited, new research has indicated that genetics has a stronger influence than we recently believed. Thomas Bouchard and his colleagues at the University of Minnesota conducted a long-term study on more than one hundred sets of identical twins who had been separated at infancy and reared apart and found that about 70 percent of the variance in IQ was associated with genetic variation. Furthermore, they found that on multiple measures of personality and temperament, occupational and leisure-time activities and social attitudes, identical twins reared apart were about as similar as identical twins reared together. Although all of these data indicate the strong influence genetics has on a wide range of traits, rather than discounting the effects of environment, the researchers hypothesized that a particular gene or set of genes most likely determines how an individual will react to his or her environment.

However we interpret these findings, once it is possible to actually control the genetic composition of one's child according to one's desires, preembryos will be selected not just because they are free of disease-causing or disease-predisposing genes, but because they possess certain characteristics we wish to perpetuate.

This new dimension will attract couples who are fertile but have failed to produce a preembryo from their own sperm and eggs with characteristics they find desirable; they can now adopt an egg, or sperm, or both.

The ultimate separation between sex and reproduction will occur by 2020 when in vitro fertilization will start a process that will continue as in vitro gestation. When that day arrives it will be possible for a baby to go from conception to birth totally outside the human body.

The advance that will make this possible will be the development of the extracorporeal gestator, or artificial placenta. A fetus developing in an artificial placenta will be watched and monitored directly rather than indirectly, as is done in the uterus. This will be especially valuable if something unexpected happens and fetal surgery needs to be performed.

Technically, an artificial placenta is not farfetched at all. According to Dr. Stephen Corson, director of the Philadelphia Fertility Clinic and clinical professor of obstetrics and gynecology at the University of Pennsylvania School of Medicine, "The main function of an artificial placenta will be to bring in nutrients and remove waste products, as does the human placenta. Since we already have heart-lung machines that accomplish a similar purpose, an artificial placenta is not at all out of the realm of possibility. But it will take about thirty years to develop."

What are we to make of all this? Obviously, the reproductive process, from conception to birth, will be a completely different phenomenon from the one we now take for granted. And each of these scientific advances is certain to generate a wide array of ethical challenges. But human nature will still have the last word. It will still be the environment in which these children of tomorrow are raised that will determine whether the selected genes flourish or wither.

# 2

# The Gardening of the Body

IF THE HUMAN SOUL AND SPIRIT ARE IMMORTAL, AS MANY OF US believe, then they are our only components that come with an extended warranty. Our tangible body parts have no warranty at all. They break, they become diseased, and usually their failure ends up causing our demise.

We've had to deal with this dilemma for thousands of years, ever since we evolved into a distinguishable species. And until very recently, we haven't dealt with it very well. If primitive man lost a limb—probably not an uncommon occurrence—he undoubtedly did without. If he escaped his predators long enough to incur a diseased organ, he quickly died. Millennia later, the only improvements were minimal and barely functional, such as wooden legs and crutches for loss of extremities. Those with diseased kidneys, livers, hearts and lungs still died without ever having had a moment's hope of recovery.

This prevailed until a half century ago. Today, the sight of a runner completing a marathon on an artificial leg or a brave four-year-old lying in a hospital bed awaiting a heart transplant pays tribute to the indomitable human spirit, but also to science for creating these opportunities. What greater testimony to twentieth-century technology is there than the ability to replace irreparably damaged or diseased body parts?

For all our successes, however, we must still be considered beginners. The athlete with the artificial limb takes three to four times as long to cover the same distance as a runner with two normal legs. The child who receives the heart transplant must take drugs to stave off the rejection of the organ his immune system so desperately wants to achieve, rendering him exposed to a variety of life-threatening infections.

The science of body part replacement is advancing so rapidly that today's technology will soon be as outdated as a wooden leg. We are on the verge of an explosion of options that most of us would have thought almost too extraordinary even for an Isaac Asimov novel, yet they are soon going to be a part of our everyday reality. A pooling of knowledge of immunologists, surgeons, molecular biologists, geneticists, gerontologists and biomedical engineers is going to result in an inexhaustible supply of natural and synthetic body parts that will replace diseased organs, avoid every transplantation-related difficulty and even replace age-worn organs and other components. And eventually this technology, too, is going to enter the realm of enhancement therapy and change the way we perform and look. Just as the application of in vitro fertilization technology is going to expand our choices before birth, the mass production of body parts is going to expand them after birth.

Prior to 1983, transplantation of healthy organs to replace diseased ones was technically possible, but not practically feasible. The barrier that could not be overcome stemmed from the fact that unless the donor and recipient were genetically—and therefore immunologically—identical, the recipient's immune surveillance cells would quickly set in motion a search and destroy mission that would result in rejection of the newly transplanted organ.

In the late 1970s, though, scientists from the Sandoz Corporation, the Swiss pharmaceutical giant, discovered that an unusual Norwegian mold (a distant cousin of the material that in an earlier generation had yielded penicillin) possessed magical properties: it was able to suppress the immune rejection response that caused most organ transplants to fail. In 1983, after several years of research and refinement, Sandoz introduced the drug cyclosporine A, which quickly became the penicillin of transplantation, creating lifesaving opportunities for tens of thousands of people.

But for many thousands more, cyclosporine A also created life-ending disappointments. The demand for organs rapidly outstripped the supply, and by 1990, in the United States alone, there were more than twenty thousand people on an ever-lengthening waiting list. Potential recipients wear electronic pagers twenty-four hours a day, waiting for the phone call that most of them never receive.

Now let's look ahead. It is 1997 and a sixty-eight-year-old retired farmer in North Dakota has reached the final stages of hypertensive kidney disease. Although he has worked hard all his life, his farm is small and the winter wheat crop often fails. He barely subsists on government largess: Social Security and Medicare. Hemodialysis is an expensive option that isn't open to him. But an inexpensive transplant procedure will save his life.

If this scenario were played out five years earlier, in 1992, the farmer would be sentenced to death. The short supply of kidneys for transplant and the toll that even the best antirejection drugs would take on his frail immune system would have eliminated him as an organ recipient candidate, as it would have almost anyone over the age of sixty.

But, in 1997, the tragedy does not take place. The farmer's physician draws a blood sample and sends it overnight seventy miles away to Fargo, the nearest medical center where his immunological tissue type can be determined. As soon as the physician has the results in hand, he faxes them, and other pertinent medical information, to the regional transplant center in Chicago. Within one hour, a cadaver match is found for the farmer.

In 1997, the shortage of cadaver organs will be markedly alleviated by the institution of a national policy of "presumed consent." Unless before death the deceased specifically prohibits the harvesting of his or her organs, or unless the family does so after death, the hospital will legally be allowed to use them.

The methods of organ preservation will also have advanced considerably. Paramedics and doctors at small community hospitals will be equipped with ice-cold blood substitutes, which will allow the organs of the deceased to be kept viable until they can be transferred to specialized transplant facilities where the organs will be removed for extended storage. Once removed from the body, instead of being kept in a viable state for just a few hours, kidneys, livers, hearts, lungs, pancreases and corneas will be indefinitely preserved in newly developed solutions, deeply frozen until needed by a compatible recipient.

The farmer in our example flies to Chicago, checks into the hospital and the transplant is successfully performed two days later. The transplant surgeon and immunologist confer and decide that this patient should take a combination of FK506 and rapamycin, two recently introduced antirejection drugs that are far more powerful than the previous miracle drug cyclosporine A. Each of these drugs works on different, specific areas of the immune response, "molecular scalpels" according to Dr. Randall Morris, director of the Laboratory for Transplantation Immunology at Stanford University Medical School. Together, they will increase the length of survival of the transplanted kidney in its new body. In addition, because of their enhanced specificity, the drugs are much gentler on the immune system, and will be well tolerated by the elderly farmer. All the new advances make organ transplantation a much more affordable reality than hemodialysis, and the entire procedure is covered by Medicare.

A forty-year-old woman in New York, a successful and wealthy real estate broker, with chronic glomerulonephritis—a progressive inflammation of the kidney that is often terminal—also needs a kidney. Unlike Medicare, this woman's insurance does not entitle her to a cadaver kidney. But she will exercise another option. She will buy a kidney from a live donor on the open market.

By 1997, body parts will have become genuine capital—the buying and selling of live donor organs will be perfectly legal and strictly regulated. Several years earlier, physicians, biomedical ethicists and the courts all will have agreed that, since a black market already existed and provided as many as 20 percent of live donor transplants, and since the organ shortage was reaching desperate proportions, the only prudent approach would be to make the selling of live donor organs legal. This practice was condoned more than ten years earlier in poorer countries such as India, where there were neither the facilities nor the technology for organ preservation. And in more developed countries, renewable body products—blood, blood components, sperm, eggs—were sold and surrogates "rented" their wombs. Legalizing the industry would eliminate unscrupulous organ brokers, who charge exorbitant fees and pocket much of the money.

The realtor's attorney, who specializes in transplant law, acts as the intermediary between her and potential anonymous voluntary donors, located through a computerized national network. The most compatible willing donor is a custodian who lives in Houston and who will sell his kidney for thirty thousand dollars, plus surgeon's and attorney's fees and administrative fees levied by the National Organ Procurement Agency, the governmental body that regulates and approves all such transactions. Immunological and financial information on the donor and recipient, along with a signed statement by the donor's physician that the donor is in good health and can medically afford to donate the kidney, is submitted by the woman's attorney to the National Organ Procurement Agency. When the go-ahead is given, surgeons in Houston remove the donor's left kidney, which is immediately preserved in Viaspan or TransTime solutions, two of the new long-life organ preservatives, slowly frozen to minus 170 degrees centigrade and shipped in that condition to the hospital in New York where the recipient will receive her kidney. Stable organ preservation removes the element of urgency from the situation, and the patient and her surgeon schedule the procedure for early the following week, after which she begins to take a combination of antirejection drugs that are similar to, but slightly different from, those taken by the North Dakota farmer.

Although the entire procedure has cost this patient more than forty-five thousand dollars and only the medical fees are covered by her insurance, she will be compensated another way. Those who buy organs and are certified to need them for lifesaving purposes but whose income is too high to qualify them for the free cadaver program will be given a hefty tax deduction.

Naturally, the only organs originating from live donors will be those that are paired (kidneys) or those capable of regenerating (a liver), in which latter case only a segment of the organ will be given to the recipient, with no danger to the health of the donor. Despite policies that will increase availability of cadaver organs, there will be a need for an additional source of hearts, lungs, pancreases and other organs.

By the year 2000, or shortly thereafter, the number one source will be xenografts—organs from nonhuman species. In 1964 Dr. Thomas Starzl, a transplantation pioneer at the University of Pittsburgh School of Medicine, kept a patient alive for six months with a chimpanzee kidney, a remarkable achievement considering the lack of sophisticated drugs to manipulate the immune system. And we all remember Baby Fay and the baboon heart in 1984. Although she didn't survive very long, both of these incidents indicated that xenografts are technically possible.

Nonhuman primates will be used routinely as a source of hearts, lungs and pancreases, and there will be colonies of them bred just for the purpose of providing these organs. The new antirejection drugs will be so potent, they will allow for immunological compatibility between humans and chimps or baboons. The use of animals so closely related to us will undoubtedly cause great ethical controversy, but another source will appear shortly after the turn of the century that will cause far greater outrage.

Anencephalic infants—babies born without a cerebral cortex—are a rarity, but they will provide the basis for a startling breakthrough. By 1997 the ethical controversy surrounding the use of their tissues for transplantation will be largely resolved. Presumed consent laws will not apply, but the majority of parents will allow these babies' organs to be used, letting some good come from a dreadful situation. Although anencephalic infants won't be a significant source, the use of their organs will provide the technical beginning for an amazing solution. But before we see what that is, let's look further at how the problem of immunological incompatibility and rejection will be resolved, since an increased supply of organs will not mean much unless we can successfully handle the threat of rejection and life-threatening infection.

By the year 2002, transplantation perfection will be reached. According to Dr. Robert Good, an immunological pioneer internationally renowned for more than thirty years, scientists are now working on something that "within ten years is going to revolutionize transplantation." Complete compatibility between donor and recipient will be achieved without the use of the double-edged sword, immunosuppressant drugs.

The technology that will be responsible for this breakthrough is the induction of immunological tolerance in adults. During fetal life, our developing immune systems learn to be "tolerant" of our own tissues so that when the immune system has fully matured, the T-cells and other policemen won't treat our tissues as foreign invaders and attack them (autoimmune diseases such as rheumatoid arthritis and multiple sclerosis are aberrations of this developmental lesson—our immune systems become intolerant of our tissues and begin to wage war on them).

In theory, if we exposed a future organ recipient to the tissues of a future donor during fetal development, the immune systems would be made tolerant of each other. Then, if the need for a transplant were to arise, the donor and the recipient would be able to exchange tissues without fear of rejection. But since we can't predict years in advance who will need an organ transplant, this is not a practical solution. What we need is a way to start the same thing happening between adults.

The day when that will be accomplished is not far off. Dr. David Sachs, former chief of immunology at the National Cancer Institute and now director of the Transplantation Biology Research Center at Massachusetts General Hospital, has been working on this for some time and is confident we will be doing exactly that by 2000.

A few weeks before receiving an organ transplant the recipient will go through a series of preparatory steps in the hospital. First, he or she will be treated with an injection of monoclonal antibodies which will directly bombard and destroy most of the T-lymphocytes, the immune system cells that are responsible for recognizing tissues as self or foreign. This will be followed by low-dose radiation to destroy any other potentially reactive T-cells in the bone marrow, the location from which the immune cells originate. All that will then be left of the recipient's potentially reactive cells will be the immunologically uncommitted "stem cells," with no preconceived notion of self from foreign. In effect, this procedure recreates a fetal immune system.

A sample of the donor bone marrow will then be taken—either aspirated from the hip of a living donor or taken from the deep freeze if the patient is to receive a cadaver organ. It too will be treated with monoclonal antibodies, again leaving only immunologically uncommitted stem cells. The treated donor bone marrow will be injected into the future recipient and the new immune system—now a mixture of donor and recipient cells—will be allowed to remature over a few-week period, developing tolerance to both donor and recipient tissues. A kidney, or any other donor organ, can be transplanted into the recipient, and it will be accepted as if it were the original. There will be absolutely no possibility that the organ will ever be rejected.

By 2002, gene transfer techniques will be perfected to the point where tolerance before transplantation will be controlled even further. Bone marrow cells will be removed from both the recipient and the donor and the uncommitted stem cells of the future recipient identified by monoclonal antibodies. Then, using an inactivated retrovirus—an agent that can act as a vehicle to transfer genes from one cell to another but which can't replicate itself— the donor genes that determine acceptance or rejection of a transplant will be transferred from the T-cells of the donor into the uncommitted stem cells of the recipient and reinjected into the recipient. After a few months, the same tolerance will be achieved.

The phenomenon of tolerance will be so well understood and the techniques so well perfected that by 2002 it will be used for xenograft transplantations as well. Human immune systems will be engineered to fully accept animal tissues without the necessity for immunosuppressive drugs. And since it will be possible to extend further across species lines, the primary source of organs will be animals raised for food consumption, such as pigs, cows and sheep.

However, as scientifically feasible as the "commodity" approach to the use of organs and animal tissues will be, the application of these discoveries will not be widespread. Government programs administering organ transactions on the open market will encounter great difficulties, and still newer solutions will evolve. And this brings us to anencephalic infants, mentioned earlier, and a bizarre scenario.

Rather than use cadaver organs or buy them on the market, by 2002 we will combine the technique of in vitro fertilization with induction of tolerance, and we will see people intentionally "creating" anencephalic infants as a source of organs for their own bodies.

A woman's egg will be fertilized in vitro with her partner's sperm and the preembryo implanted in a chimpanzee uterus. After six weeks, a surgeon will remove the fetus and cut away the primitive brain cells (and freeze for later use if needed). Then the fetus will be reimplanted into the chimp and allowed to develop to term. At the end of the nine-month gestation period, a "human vegetable" will be born, a brainless and soulless repository of fully functioning organs. Since the genetic structure of the tissues will be derived half from the man and half from the woman, it will be a simple matter to induce tolerance to whoever needs the transplant. The not quite human baby will be either kept alive on a life-support system or frozen, depending on how soon the transplant will be performed.

Another development, which will make us considerably less uncomfortable to imagine, will begin about 2000 when we start to see the routine use of totally implantable artificial organs. At first, they will appear cumbersome and operate inefficiently, the beneficiaries of this technology encumbered by battery packs worn 354at the waist and by the frequent malfunctioning. Later though, by 2010, all regulatory elements will be internal and totally hidden from view. This will be more than a cosmetic improvement. The perfected implantable body parts will function as well as, and in many cases better than, the real thing.

In some patients implantation will totally replace transplantation, eliminating the need for natural organ transplants all together. In other patients there will be a mix of biological organs and synthetically created ones. And as the science progresses even further, these human-machine combinations will be not only within one body but within individual organs. Rather than replace an entire pancreas, for example, only the insulin-secreting beta cells will be implanted, leaving the remainder of the organ biologically intact.

Initial uses of artificial body part technology will be to help the sick, but that will be a mere prelude to a whole host of enhancement therapies that will grow as fast as we can think up innovations.

We had a brief, not very successful fling with artificial organs in the 1980s. Dr. Robert Jarvik, the developer of the artificial heart, and Barney Clark, his patient, were pioneers, but the thinking was ahead of the technology of the day. Because of a variety of complications (primarily strokes in the recipients), the Food and Drug Administration banned the Jarvik heart in 1989.

Recently, and without much fanfare, there has been a resurgence and some impressive progress in the field of artificial organs. One of the leaders is Dr. Daniel Schneck, whose credentials—he is a pathologist and a biomedical engineer—make him uniquely equipped to develop replacement body parts. At his laboratory in the hills of Blacksburg, Virginia, he and his colleagues at Virginia Polytechnic Institute have applied what they've learned from their work on the design of space stations to ideas about the manufacture of totally implantable artificial organs.

The materials for a space station must be efficient, nontoxic to the environment and lightweight, and the parts microminiature—all criteria necessary for artificial organs. In order to compensate for the effects of the near-zero-gravity space environment, biomedical engineers have also had to learn a tremendous amount about human physiology. They have stripped down the operation of the body into pure engineering principles—the human body as a finely tuned electrochemical engine, one that takes in fuel, distributes it, metabolizes it and eliminates the waste. As a result of what they have learned, engineers are designing synthetic organs that are efficient and cheap.

In order for the engineered organs to function, they will first have to live in harmony with our bodies. Just as our immune system will reject a nongenetically identical human organ, so will it mount a similar attack against a foreign body part made of synthetic materials. The solution is going to come from the Human Genome Project. By 2005, when it is completed, we will know the structure of every one of the 100,000 human genes, including those that determine immunological compatibility. Using that information, it will then be possible to endow synthetic materials with biological properties, and totally implantable organs will become a practical reality.

Implantation will be much different from transplantation. For one thing, the entire procedure will eventually be handled mostly on an outpatient basis. In 2010, when patients need an artificial heart, they won't have to try to make do with a cadaver organ or one from an animal, or to create their own anencephalic vegetable. Instead, their doctor will write them a prescription for an artificial heart, which they will take to their local Radio Shack or other electronic store. From the human technology section, they will purchase their new heart right off the shelf. Although the organs won't, of course, be one size fits all—there will be different models for children and adults—neither will they have to be custom-made. Each one will contain biosensors fitted with microchips which, when implanted, will be able to monitor a variety of physiological functions. And through feedback mechanisms, the input-output controls will be automatically adjusted. A 230-pound man will need greater cardiac output than a 115-pound woman, yet with the appropriate sensors the same heart will be capable of adapting to either of them. And it will also be able to adapt to varying needs within the same person, automatically adjusting to the differences between a sedentary body and one engaged in athletics.

The person who buys the artificial heart will then take it to an implantation laboratory, an elaborate facility with high-speed gene sequencers, mainframe computers with computer-aided design (CAD) capability and a storehouse of synthetic materials. A blood sample will be drawn and the future recipient sent home, to report to the affiliated implantation clinic one week later.

In the interim, the patient's DNA will be analyzed on a gene sequencer, and a computer will then discern the geometric structure of the HLA (human leukocyte antigen) gene, an immunological marker that determines tissue compatibility. The CAD computer will design a geometric structure that exactly duplicates that of the patient's HLA. Synthetic materials will then be used to create that structure, after which it will be mixed with biopolymers that will coat the surface of the artificial heart, especially at the interface between synthetic and natural tissue, providing the heart with the genetic-immunological properties of the patient.

During the several days the heart is being prepared for implantation, the patient goes to the physiology section of the implant clinic and has a noninvasive cardiac output study performed. Because his own heart doesn't function well enough for him to perform an exercise test, the computer deduces what his maximum output would need to be under the most demanding of circumstances and relays this information to the laboratory. After the artificial heart has been coated with the biopolymers, the biosensor settings are fixed to conform with the physiological data derived from the natural organ.

The following week the patient returns to the implantation clinic early in the morning, where the old heart will be removed and the now-prepared artificial heart implanted. Using ice-cold technology, the operation is almost entirely bloodless, and the patient is sent home within just a few days. Although he will have a brief recuperation period, it will be in the comfort of his own home, and within a few more days he will be functioning as if he were twenty years younger.

This same scenario will be repeated for virtually every organ in the body: kidneys, livers, lungs, pancreases. In most cases, biomedical engineers will defer to millions of years of evolution and design artificial organs to mimic natural function as closely as possible. But sometimes there will be an opportunity to go Mother Nature one better.

The artificial kidney will be an example. As Dr. Schneck explained, our kidney is not designed the way an engineer would fashion an organ for waste elimination, the primary function of the kidney. The natural version of the human kidney works by first excreting all materials—those it wants to eliminate as well as those it wants to retain—through one set of tubules, and then reabsorbing the elements it wants to keep through a second set. Although the system performs elegantly, biomedical engineers will create a filtering system that eliminates the redundancy, merely excreting what isn't wanted at the first pass. The kidney we pick off the shelf in 2010 will work differently from our own, but more efficiently.

The progress in artificial body components will not be limited to production of visceral organs, but will expand to perfecting a sensory organ technology that will make available completely implantable artificial eyes and ears. As of now, the artificial eye prototypes that have been developed are quite primitive and presuppose that the optic nerve—the connection between the eye and the brain—is intact. The same is true for artificial ears, cochlear implants that must communicate with the brain through the auditory nerve. By 2015, though, the capability of artificial eyes and ears will be so far advanced they will even surpass our own.

Developing perfectly functioning sensory organs will take longer than creating a heart or kidney because the process is more complex. The sensory organs are the body's information systems, the means by which various parts communicate with each other. They are continually sending and receiving impulses to and from specific areas of the brain, in bursts called action potentials. In order to design an artificial organ with similar capabilities, not only must steps be taken to ensure immunological compatibility, but biomedical engineers must first decode this language.

Piece by piece, like the parts of the most complex jigsaw puzzle imaginable, this is being accomplished. When it is finished, there will be artificial eyes and ears that can interact physiologically with the body in terms of information transport, sending and receiving messages through the same channels and in the same way as their natural counterparts. And, in an astonishing technological advance, scientists will develop implantable artificial optic and auditory nerves—the linkage of the eyes and ears with the brain. The new sensory organs will be attached either to the existing nerve or, if it is not intact, to the artificial one which will be implanted with the organ. Blindness and deafness will be totally eliminated, a tremendous boon to everyone afflicted but especially to the elderly, who make up more than 50 percent of those either legally blind or deaf or severely impaired.

There will be artificial arms that will be able to impart a sense of touch; the arm will be interfaced with the sensory nerves and will contain pressure receptors in the fingers, just as our natural fingers do. Someone with an artificial arm implanted will be able to discriminate between objects as we can—determining the difference between a Nerf ball and a hard ball, a dime and a quarter—without looking. Besides perfect sensory capability, these arms will have complete motor function, and since they will be designed to respond to the same signals to which a natural arm does, they will move in a completely natural manner. They will even be covered with human skin, indistinguishable from our own arms in every way.

The same technology will also allow for the creation of naturally functioning artificial legs. For those who have lost a limb as the result of some traumatic accident and whose spinal cord is still intact, these artificial legs will be the hoped-for miracle. For quadriplegics and paraplegics, who still have their limbs but whose spinal columns are partially or completely transected, artificial nerves—derived from the same biomedical engineering breakthrough that will cure blindness and deafness—will be able to bypass a break in the spinal cord.

The operative procedure will be similar to the way an artery is bypassed, but more complicated, since the blood vessel graft functions essentially as a conduit for blood, whereas a nerve bypass will have to transmit and receive impulses between spinal cord and brain. But we're calling for this to be available by 2015. It's difficult to imagine anything more dramatic than a quadriplegic who today might not even be able to feed himself running and dancing as if his trauma had never been experienced.

For nerves that are not irreparably damaged, biomedical engineers are also working on ways of electromagnetically inducing natural tissue regeneration. Every time an injury is inflicted upon a part of our body, the affected part generates what is called an injury potential. By activating a cellular network around the injury, the injury potential triggers the healing process. Through engineering analysis of these biological signals, scientists are learning to duplicate them and transmit the same type of signals to an injured body part and stimulate growth and regeneration.

This has already been shown to be effective in inducing bones to heal. For fractures that heal poorly, it is possible to stimulate the bone electrically so that the osteoblasts—the bone cells responsible for growth—can be tricked into "thinking" a biological injury potential has activated them to begin healing. At the present time, there is a downside to this procedure. Any time cells are artificially "turned on," there is the potential danger that they won't know when to turn off, and the uncontrolled cell growth could lead to cancer. But, by 2010, the stimulation-activation responses will be fully elucidated and routinely used clinically.

This technique will be applied not just to recalcitrant fractures, but to speeding up the process for those that would heal normally. A fracture that under normal biological circumstances might take six weeks to heal will be healed in just one or two weeks, an advance that will have far-reaching benefits, especially for professional athletes.

These advances are going to transform our lives. But it is when we get into the area of using artificial body parts to enhance natural function that our society will be transformed.

Let's consider, for example, the human knee, so beautifully designed for walking and running. But it is not meant to be subjected to the torque stresses (twisting) imposed upon it by the rigors of other athletic endeavors, notably football, basketball and soccer. Even casual fans have heard the words "torn cruciate ligaments" enough to be familiar with the terminology and its season- or career-ending implications for their favorite athletes.

By 2010 to 2015, biomedical engineers will have perfected the artificial knee—the professional sports version. The professional knee will be designed to take a severe torque without ligaments or joint capsule tearing. Athletes will no longer have to suffer serious crippling injuries and for that reason the professional knee will become standard equipment the way shoulder pads, helmets and face guards are now. It will be prohibited in high school and college athletics but available to professionals. As long as the artificial knee is standard equipment and used by everyone, no athlete will gain an unfair advantage over another. And the artificial knee will be used primarily to prevent injuries and prolong careers, not specifically to enhance performance.

Opportunities for deceitfully enhancing performance will abound, however. Instead of having to rigorously practice plyometrics in order to jump higher, a ballet dancer or basketball player will be tempted to surreptitiously have artificial muscles and ligaments implanted that will give them more spring. Or a baseball player who dreams of a multimillion-dollar contract might want to have a synthetic eye inserted that contains more light-discriminating sensors than a natural eye and which will make him a better hitter than even Joe Hardy of *Damn Yankees* fame.

On the other hand, outside of athletics, there will be situations where an enhanced performance will be more altruistically motivated. The artificial eye that the baseball player will most likely be prohibited from using will prove desirable for prolonging the career of a skilled surgeon. And since there will be virtually complete understanding of physiological processes and interorgan communication, it will be possible to "rewire" the body any way we like. It would literally be possible to have eyes in the back of our head if we so wished.

Nothing evokes images of science fiction (or Woody Allen comedies) more than cloning, but by 2020, it is going to be the dominant body-part technology. Artificial components will still be used, but their demand will be primarily limited to enhancement functions, doing things that even perfect versions of our own organs can't. Transplantation as it exists today—and all attendant problems— will be entirely obsolete.

Significant progress has already been made in this area. As far back as the fifties, frogs were cloned from embryos, and more recently the same has been accomplished with mice, sheep, rabbits and cows. Human cloning is on the near horizon. Dr. Paul Segall of Berkeley, California, one of the leaders in this field, feels strongly we will see the first human cloned within ten years and it will be in routine clinical use within thirty.

Lest we envision the creation of multiple cookie-cutter versions of ourselves we should set our minds at ease. It won't be possible. The clones will begin from embryos and, although genetically identical with us, will be raised in a very different environment. What we are going to see is body cloning, not the creation of another living, breathing human being, but the duplication of our body parts so that we can use them at will.

By about 2020, the following scenario could take place. At the age of twenty-five or thirty, when we have physically developed to our peak, we will pay a visit to the twenty-first-century version of a cosmetic surgeon. After signing the appropriate releases, the surgeon will administer a local anesthetic and snip a small piece of skin from the underside of our arm. She will quickly drop the skin into a glass laboratory dish, in which the skin tissue will be bathed in enzymes that break it up into individual cells. Then, under a dissecting microscope, the surgeon will tease away just the nucleus from one of the skin cells and draw it up into a tiny hollow glass needle called a micropipette.

Again under the microscope, the nucleus will be injected, in another laboratory dish, into a purchased human egg cell whose own nucleus (and therefore genetic information) has been destroyed by ultraviolet light. Genetically engineered DNA that mimics the signals given to a fertilized egg will be added to stimulate this new cell to divide. The entire procedure will then be repeated exactly, using another skin cell and denucleated human egg. As is done with in vitro fertilization, the fertilized eggs will remain for a few days in a medium that contains oviduct cells from the lining of the fallopian tube. Once it has reached the size of the head of a pin, the preembryos will be implanted into a uterus to develop further. If the development of an artificial placenta keeps pace with cloning technology, that is where the preembryos will be implanted, but if perfected cloning technology antedates the artificial placenta, the womb of a great ape, such as a chimp or baboon, will be used.

In either case, the environment will have been hormonally prepared to accept the preembryos (and if it is an ape, immunologically prepared as well) before implantation. Six weeks later, the surgeon will remove the embryos and, under the microscope, dissect away the primitive cells that, if left to their own devices, would develop into a fully functioning human brain. These cells will not be discarded but frozen in liquid nitrogen to be used at a later date if needed. What will be left are not six-week-old human fetuses, but six-week old brainless and soulless humanoids, which will grow to become repositories of spare body parts.

After thirty-four more weeks, the body clones will come to full term and be delivered, either by cesarean section if developed in an ape uterus, or by simple extraction if development took place in the artificial placenta. Similar in appearance to an anencephalic infant, but genetically identical with the person from which it originated, it will be kept alive by a feeding tube. Growth and maturation will be accelerated by injections of genetically engineered hormones. After two years, the clones will be removed from their life-support systems and placed in cryonic suspension, an updated version of the same deep-freeze solution that will be used to indefinitely store organs for transplant by the end of the 1990s. There they will remain until needed, at which time they will be disassembled into their component parts as necessary, either to cure a life-threatening illness or to rejuvenate lost youth with new skin, muscles and organs. Since they will be genetically identical with us, they will be immediately accepted by our immune systems without the necessity for immunosuppressant drugs or even the biopolymer coatings needed for artificial organs. A second clone will remain as a backup so body parts will be available indefinitely. When one clone is used, the second will be temporarily thawed, used to create another backup and then refrozen.

Through genetic engineering, it will also be possible to create our cloned parts to be immunologically identical but in other ways different from the original. Before our snipped skin cells are injected into the awaiting egg, new genes can be insinuated into the DNA at the appropriate spot and comparable ones removed. If we desire blue eyes instead of brown, a cosmetic surgeon will merely switch our brown-eye gene for a blue one. Or if we want to be taller in our new incarnation, tallness genes will be added to our skin cell DNA and grow up in our body clone. When at age sixty we have our bone and muscle transplant, along with appropriate hormonal support, we will begin to grow again. Virtually any physical metamorphosis we desire will be possible.

Another technology will be available before the end of this decade and will become a prelude to cloning. Embryos begun by in vitro fertilization will be divided in two at the four-cell stage and each allowed to divide a few more times. Then one of the preembryos will be implanted in a uterus and developed into a healthy baby. The other genetically identical preembryo will be frozen.

Fifteen years later, when the technology exists for growing body clones and for storing them cryonically, the frozen preembryo will be thawed and developed as a clone to the now fifteen-year-old child. Those that begin with in vitro fertilization will in fifteen years have the luxury of growing more than one clone, allowing one clone to develop immediately as a safeguard against accident or injury (genetic engineering of preembryos will be available by this time, so congenital diseases will be eliminated), and freezing the other one for use in later life.

At first cloning will be prohibitively expensive, available only to the very wealthy. But just as with any new technology, as it develops it will become cheaper and there will be competition. Eventually it will be within the reach of many.

The combination of cloning and artificial organs will create human beings who are both physically superior and tremendously long-lived, perhaps immortal. Religious questions aside, for those of us who are concerned about exacerbation of world overpopulation, we can feel confident that the space program will be developing concomitantly and that space stations will provide the answer.

The ultimate organ to either transplant, create artificially or clone is, of course, the brain, something we have only briefly alluded to here. So important and so exciting are the developments in this area that they deserve a discussion all their own.

# 3

# Outthinking the Brain

THE STUDENT COMPLETES HER EXAM IN RECORD TIME AND WITH a near-perfect score. The grieving widower decides his time for mourning is up and it abruptly ends. The struggling artist has a planned burst of creativity. After years of unsuccessfully battling to lose weight, the obese patient begins to see the pounds melt off for good. The house-bound mother of two young children and an elderly woman experience an exciting adventure without leaving their living rooms.

These are just a few of the life-enhancing therapies we can expect to see in the next three decades. They will all come about because we are standing on the verge of conquering the last great scientific frontier: exploring and understanding the mysteries of the human brain.

Beginning with its appearance, the brain is full of surprises. Despite the labyrinth of ridges and crevices (called gyri and sulci), its landscape presents a homogeneous, almost placid appearance. The pink-tan tissue is so soft and spongy that neuropathologists must bathe the brain in a formaldehyde solution for as long as a week before being able to slice it for anatomic and microscopic study.

But the calm and passive exterior belies the incredible beehive of intense activity that takes place at our command central, an advanced neuroscientific laboratory hidden within some remote mountain cave. The billions of neurons embedded microscopically within the brain are constantly firing off mini-explosions of electrical and biochemical activity that determine virtually every facet of our being—our personality, our memory, our emotions, our creativity. Being able to decipher how all this occurs will be a scientific accomplishment of the highest order, not only unlocking the secrets of the ages, but more important opening wide boulevards to the future. Once this is done, the behavior-oriented mind control techniques of past decades will be replaced by precise biochemically oriented brain control techniques. Biochemistry will displace what we now call the mind-body relationship.

This, of course, has been something man has been pursuing for thousands of years, ever since he began contemplating the nature of his existence. But the brain has guarded its secrets jealously. The mechanisms by which it directs our lives have remained almost impervious to scientific probing.

Ignorance is often a prologue to fear. Because of our inability to comprehend the workings of the brain, those with miswired or biochemically aberrant cerebrums have been ostracized from society, often treated as criminals. Although psychiatry moved away from straitjackets and "Snake Pit" hospitals decades ago, patients with mental disorders continued to be looked upon by many physicians with curiosity and the same feeling of helplessness one had for the pneumonia victim in the days before antibiotics. Psychiatry was properly considered by most members of the medical profession to be more of an art than a science, and this assessment still holds.

But there has been a stunning change. The neurosciences, which include much of what psychiatry is all about today, are now making more progress than any other branch of medicine. Ninety percent of what we know about the brain has been learned in the past ten years, and we have barely scratched the surface. But in recognition of a new direction, President Bush and Congress have jointly proclaimed the nineties as the "decade of the brain." Little did they realize the extent of unsettling events their proclamation was anticipating.

Molecular biology and genetics are the fields that will contribute to the accelerated unraveling of brain chemistry and physiology. Through these new disciplines, virtually every previously unsolvable neuroscientific problem is going to be conquered. Nothing will escape scientific understanding.

In 1990, Dr. Solomon Snyder and his colleagues at the department of neuroscience at Johns Hopkins University School of Medicine reported that they had successfully cultured human brain cells in the laboratory. Although the implications of this were not evident to most of us at the time, it was a major breakthrough. It meant that neuroscientists now had the tool all other biological scientists have deemed crucial to research—a human cell line on which to experiment. This, along with key discoveries in neurochemistry, is providing a springboard for expanding our knowledge of how the brain functions and malfunctions, how it interacts with the rest of the body, how we think, how we dream, how we have visions, and how we remember.

Not only will the research provide insights and progress into the treatment of many of the neurodegenerative and psychiatric diseases, such as Alzheimer's disease, Parkinson's disease and schizophrenia, but it will have an impact on how we all live our lives. On demand, we will be able to safely and effectively manipulate our emotions. We will be able to supplant anxiety, hatred, fear, pain and helplessness with confidence, love, pleasure and creativity. Our lives will be filled with higher peaks than ever before, and without the deep valleys too many of us experience. Not only will disease and age-related memory loss be obliterated, but memory enhancement of several orders of magnitude will be possible. The brain as a computer will finally be used as we now use our desktops and laptops.

As with all the scientific and medical advances we are going to witness in the next few decades, the impetus will come from the need to understand and treat disease. From there, though, it will be just a few short biochemical steps toward using this knowledge to enhance the lives of the healthy.

Many people believe that the widespread occurrence of drug addiction presents the single greatest health problem that society will have to deal with in the next twenty years. But Dr. Julius Axelrod, Nobel laureate in medicine and the recipient of the first Neuroscience Achievement Award, depicts an alternate scenario, in which the addiction dilemma is reduced to a minor problem. We will soon understand the primary reason for all forms of addiction, and the solution won't be social or political or military, but biochemical.

We made a giant step forward in 1990 when Dr. Ernest Noble, professor of alcohol studies and director of the Alcohol Research Center at UCLA School of Medicine, together with his California colleagues and scientists at the University of Texas at San Antonio, discovered the gene for alcoholism. Similar breakthroughs will isolate the genes for other forms of addiction—from drugs to nicotine to food—and out of all this will come, in the proper sequence, specific and highly effective treatments for the addiction, followed by an effective preventive therapy.

But it won't be just addicts who will benefit from this rational and targeted treatment and prevention. What we are going to learn about normal brain biochemistry from the development of these treatments is going to change the daily lives of ordinary people.

Imagine this: It is 1997 and a twenty-five-year-old man is arrested for the second time in a six-month period for driving while intoxicated, the breathalyzer test showing more than twice the legal limit on each occasion. In order to have his driver's license reinstated, he must be willing to go through certain tests at the alcohol treatment center. He confers with his physician, who tells him that the test he will take will result in him either getting his license back shortly or, perhaps, having it permanently revoked.

At the treatment center, he fills out a detailed personality questionnaire and submits to psychological and brain wave tests. Then a technician comes to take a vial of blood. By use of the same polymerase chain reaction that is going to be so important in other areas of medicine, the DNA is separated from the rest of the cellular material, cut by enzymes to isolate a specific segment and that segment then amplified billions of times. Molecular probes are then used to detect the presence or absence of an alcohol-predisposing gene—and this is what makes the anecdote important.

But now we've got to realize that the so-called gene for alcoholism isn't really that at all; there are so many complex environmental factors involved in becoming addicted to alcohol or any other substance that genetics doesn't always play a part. If exposed enough, anyone will become addicted to a habituating substance. Nevertheless, there *is* something in the makeup of those who become addicts that almost preordains their addiction. For them, using and abusing drugs becomes an almost irresistible seduction. And the genetics and molecular biology of that "something" are what will eventually affect us all.

Here's how it works. In our brain, there is a set of neurons called the nucleus accumbens that comprise the "pleasure center." On the surface of these neurons, as on the surface of all brain cells, there are receptors for a variety of neurotransmitters, the chemical messengers by which brain cells communicate with each other. In order for a message to be conveyed from one cell to another, the neurotransmitter must first anchor itself firmly to the receptor and then signal to the inside of the cell to respond in a certain way, depending on what message is being sent.

Like a lock and key, each of the receptors will allow only a specific neurotransmitter to attach. The neurotransmitter that is perhaps the number one stimulator of our pleasure center is called dopamine, a chemical that has several other functions in our body as well. Every day, we have many pleasurable experiences, the little things that make our lives enjoyable: a warm shower on a cold morning, a stimulating conversation, a good hard game of tennis, making love, reading an exciting book. What happens biochemically when we are experiencing these delights is that a stream of the neurotransmitter dopamine is released and these molecules attach to their specific receptor on the surface of the cells in our pleasure center, setting off a constellation of electrical and biochemical activity that we interpret as pleasure.

The alcoholic, on the other hand—at least 25 to 30 percent of those Dr. Noble has studied—isn't so fortunate. An accident of genetics has left him with a structurally abnormal receptor as well as fewer of them. When he performs a job well, or listens to Beethoven's Ninth Symphony, he doesn't get the same pleasurable experience the rest of us do. Dopamine is released, but since it doesn't fit perfectly into the receptor on the pleasure center, the message doesn't get through to the brain that this is something to be enjoyed. It's not an all-or-none phenomenon, but the pleasure these people feel is much less than what someone with a normal dopamine receptor experiences. The small pleasures of everyday living are not going to provide enough positive feelings to offset or compensate for a normal dose of aggravation. A drink will be needed to get those positive feelings to flow.

Imagine living virtually all your life with no significant external stimulation of your pleasure center. These are the alcoholics. We will now refer to them as having abnormal pleasure-seeking genes. Alcohol is such a powerful stimulant of the dopamine receptor that, even though it poorly fits the body's needs, the pleasure message gets through. The key may not fit the lock—but it manages to down the door.

Although Dr. Noble and his colleagues have so far found the abnormal receptor in only about one quarter to one third of the alcoholics they studied, and in those with specific personality and neuropsychological characteristics, their research is getting a big boost from molecular biology. Whereas just a few years ago, the specific configuration of any dopamine receptors was unknown, now scientists are finding that there are many subtypes of them. At the rate progress is being made, within five years other abnormal dopamine receptor subtypes will be identified. Within ten years we will understand the differences between the genetic predispositions to alcohol and cocaine addiction.

There are whole classes of other neurochemicals in the brain, each with their own receptors that can go wrong. By 2005, abnormal serotonin and norepinephrine receptors will be found to be involved in heroin addiction, nicotine addiction, obesity and sugar-cravings.

Returning to our scenario of the twenty-five-year-old man arrested for drunk driving, we see that the molecular probe determines that he does indeed have an abnormal dopamine receptor gene, and unfortunately it is the gene that predisposes to the most severe kind of alcoholism. The allure of drinking for this patient is so strong that there is statistically less than a 20 percent chance he will be able to remain sober for long periods. His driver's license is revoked.

Meanwhile another patient arrested under the same circumstances is found to have a different genetic abnormality, one that does not predispose her to as severe a form of alcoholism. Her license is merely suspended for three months while she undergoes behavioral therapy.

Since, in 1997, there won't be any drugs available to take advantage of this newly gained biochemical knowledge, it is by no means an ideal situation. But the classification of alcoholics into different genetic categories is the beginning of a new and useful therapy based on molecular biology, a major shift from the supportive and behavioral emphasis of today. It is a perfect example of how the medicine of the future is going to be individualized.

Five years later, by 2002, the pharmaceutical and biotechnology industries will have entered the picture and changed the outcome of these molecular diagnoses. Based on the information discovered about the various subtypes of abnormal dopamine receptors, computers will be employed to design small dopaminelike molecules to conform to the shape of the abnormally configured receptors. These will then be synthesized into compounds that, when swallowed, will be absorbed into the bloodstream and carried into the spinal fluid that bathes the brain. They will attach to the abnormal receptors as tightly as naturally made dopamine would to the normal dopamine receptors. There will be different compounds to react with each of the different kinds of abnormal receptors, only slight differences in molecular structure making all the difference in the activation of the pleasure center. Patients will take these specially designed compounds every day, as "vitamins" for their brain's pleasure center. Doing so will bring these people up to the neurochemical level of the rest of us. People who are arrested for DWI won't have to lose their driving privileges at all. They will willingly take their medication every day because these drugs will make them feel good, something they won't ever have experienced before without the strong stimulus of alcohol. And because the compounds are so specifically designed, they will cause no side effects at all. These people will be completely cured of their alcoholism, as long as they continue to take the drugs.

By 2005 there will be medications for all other forms of addiction. Since all the different receptor subtypes will have been genetically identified, different "brain vitamins" will be designed to replace the stimulus of cocaine and heroin, and addicts will be extricated from the life-choking drug trap. Since these nonaddicting medications will be so effective, there will be no need for interdiction or other expenses of the present-day drug programs. The substances will be entirely underwritten by the government and distributed free in schools throughout the country, especially in the inner cities. The effect on society will be staggering. Crime rates will plummet precipitously, domestic and foreign drug lords will disappear and scores of inner-city kids will finally have a legitimate chance at success.

The design of biochemicals to fit tightly into the nicotine receptors on the brain cells will at last provide us with the smokeless society we have been working toward. As a result of not smoking, at least one thousand lives per day will be saved, and the health care system will, in turn, save billions of dollars.

Another problem, obesity, resembles an addiction in that the brain plays a prominent role in most cases. In a certain region of the brain (the hypothalamus) there are both a satiety center and an appetite center. The interaction of these centers with a variety of neurotransmitters—GABA, cholecystokinin, dynorphin, neuropeptide Y—signals us to eat or not to eat. As with other brain functions, the messages must be delivered through receptors, all of which are subject to genetic perturbations.

In addition, female sex hormones play a role. Because of the interaction of estrogen and progesterone with the neurotransmitter receptors, women who inherit the same genetic abnormality that would predispose a man to either alcoholism or cocaine addiction will be more prone to overeating, which, social factors notwithstanding, helps explain why obesity is more common in women.

By 2005, an explosion of research in this area will revolutionize the way in which obesity is treated, dramatically improving the outcome. Obesity clinics will first draw blood from new patients and test for genetic abnormalities in neurotransmitter receptor function. Depending on the results of the analysis, synthetic compounds will be administered that will either enhance the fit between an appetite-suppressing neurotransmitter and its receptor or antagonize the interaction between an appetite-stimulating neurotransmitter and its receptor. Exercise and diet will still be mainstays of any weight management program, but the group of patients who, no matter how hard they try can't lose weight, will for the first time become thin and stay thin.

These scenarios are not meant to depict some future biochemical land of Oz, a fantasy world where everyone lives a happy, productive, completely trouble-free life, but rather to indicate the scientific potential for relegating so many societal ills to the trash heap of the past. All of these treatments will be analogous to the therapy of the most common type of diabetes, in which patients have either too few or improperly functioning receptors for insulin on the surface of their cells. The diet, drugs or nutrients these people use are meant to improve receptor function, the exact same approach that will be used with addiction of all kinds.

Beginning in 2005, the same treatments directed at altering the brain chemistry of the addict will be applied to preventing addiction from the outset. Before beginning school, children will be given a mandatory blood test so that the genetic composition of their brain receptors can be analyzed. The tests themselves will be cheap and the application of the results will save billions of dollars. Before they are ever exposed to drugs or nicotine, it will be determined whether young children have any genetic abnormality that will make them more prone to addiction. An appropriate safe, synthetic substitute, which will stimulate their pleasure centers the same way some dangerous addicting compound would, will be administered, eliminating a need to use an addicting substance.

The success of these preventive programs in those with a genetic aberration will lead to their use with children who have no genetic abnormalities in their neurotransmitter receptors at all but who still might seek heightened pleasure through drugs or alcohol. These kids will be given good drugs instead, substances of virtue and no adversity. They will be administered daily in schools in all disadvantaged neighborhoods, in the cafeteria with the noon meal. As with compounds used for treatment of various addictions, since these products will generate feelings of mild euphoria, there won't be any resistance to taking them, and this will guarantee their overall success.

It is essential to understand that we are not talking about "happy pills." These new drugs will eradicate whatever blocks we experience in responding to normal positive stimuli—the familiar everyday things that make life agreeable. This is the "euphoria" we're seeking. A kid who's in a miserable environment or one who's being abused won't suddenly be "tricked" into thinking everything's rosy. That would be fascistic and evil; and it's not in the cards.

The elderly are a group ready-made for a similar program: retired, perhaps widowed, and often cut off from the stimulation of meaningful daily contact. Advertisements for retirement communities in Florida and other warm climates promise permanent "good times," a way to live out one's remaining days in happiness and peace. By 2010, though, older citizens will have another option. Instead of moving to Florida to experience pleasure, they will be able to get a daily dose of it at home in Montana or Minnesota or wherever. The routine use of these synthetic substances by elderly people living independently as well as those in nursing homes will eliminate feelings of depression and loneliness—and will give them a chance to interact with other people whose company they will still require. The need for social programs will not be eliminated, but the benefits of a good program will be enhanced.

These euphoria drugs will bear no resemblance to present-day antidepressants, crude by comparison in their psychopharmacological effects and with a multitude of side effects. Nor will these substances induce a state of permanent ecstasy, where the elderly shuffle about in a zombielike pleasure stupor. Behavior will not be noticeably altered, except that those who take the euphoric compounds will be capable of enjoying the same daily pleasures as they did when they were younger.

The day will come—we're calling for it by around 2015—when this concept is taken one logical step further, the application of this research to those who are neither genetically nor environmentally disadvantaged but who will have the opportunity to fine-tune their lives in supernormal fashion. By then it will be possible not just to safely induce a feeling of euphoria but to selectively amplify or blunt virtually every emotion and feeling we experience. Many experts have concluded that we use at most 10 percent of our brain power, not just of memory but creativity and imagination. Being able to unleash some of this will have the potential to tremendously enhance our lives.

September 3, 2021. Alexa, an attractive twenty-six-year-old junior associate at a prestigious law firm, sits on the commuter train contemplating her big moment—today she is trying her first case. Ever since she was in her early teens, she has wanted to be a trial lawyer and, up to now, seems to be right on track toward realizing her childhood dream. She came to her position with stellar credentials, having graduated third in her class at the University of Chicago Law School, in addition to being editor of the law review. But unknown to everyone except those closest to her, Alexa has a problem: a fear of speaking to groups, by her definition any gathering of more than two people. She intellectually knows the cause of her difficulty—a lack of confidence "instilled" in her by her father, for whom no performance in academics, swimming or the flute (all of which she excelled in) was ever quite good enough. But knowing why she lacks confidence is not enough. Being the determined and bright woman she is, she has usually managed to mask this anxiety, but Alexa suffers terribly the night before even minor presentations, and knows that it keeps her from doing her best. No matter how well prepared she is, she invariably feels a warm flush on the back of her neck as she begins to speak, her neurochemical signal that her fear is manifesting itself again. Knowing the law and how to apply it won't be enough for her to be successful; a distinguished trial attorney must also be an actor of sorts, able to perform confidently in front of a group.

Finally, Alexa decides to reveal to a physician this secret, her glaring shortcoming. Admitting this to anyone outside her intimate circle takes real resolve, but she realizes she will never attain the level of success she desires without help.

Alexa's physician finds her insightful and engaging and spends almost two hours discussing the details of her problem with her. Eventually he agrees with her—the problem is a lack of confidence. A blood test is taken and one week later Alexa is told that she has no genetic abnormalities in neurotransmitter receptor function that could be contributing to her predictable reaction. The situation is purely environmental, her father being the culprit. Her doctor writes a prescription for a specific stimulant of the subtype of norepinephrine receptor closely associated with generating feelings of confidence. At first Alexa balks; it might be better to stay with uncomfortable, yet familiar feelings rather than risk some unknown side effects that might make her too tranquil, or worse, cause her to be even less confident. However, her physician assures her that no such thing will happen. She will be as mentally sharp as before the drug, with an even keener edge because the feelings and signs of lack of confidence won't be there to interfere. Within thirty minutes of taking the drug and for ninety minutes thereafter, there will be a controlled shower of neurochemical reactions that will make Alexa feel exactly as she would want to before a presentation—calm, confident and collected. The drug won't do the preparation for her but it will allow her to most effectively demonstrate what she has prepared.

The development of such effective pharmacological means of modulating behavior is going to make psychotherapy obsolete. We won't need to spend countless hours and dollars in self-flagellating analysis or behavior-modification exercises. The results will be there when we want them and be completely effective. Conditions and situations, such as Alexa's, for which most of us wouldn't even think of consulting a psychotherapist, will be handled easily. Every emotion or feeling we experience is the result of a biochemical reaction in our brain. Psychotherapy is a crude attempt to affect biochemistry by controlling the stimulus of the reaction. In the future, we will go straight to the heart of the matter and control the biochemical pathway itself.

Having "whited out" four canvases in a row, George is becoming both aggravated and despondent. All during his training at the Art Institute he was told he has enormous artistic talent but that he has to learn to get more in touch with his creativity, to let his mind and feelings guide his brushstrokes. But it has been an agonizing three years for George. He has only produced two inferior paintings, and both he and his mentor are frustrated. It's not nearly up to his potential. Often George feels as if he has the vision of what he wants to paint clearly in his mind, but it is so fleeting he can't capture it long enough to translate to the canvas.

George's mentor, a philanthropist and elder statesman of the art world who relishes discovering and nurturing new talent, arranges an appointment for him with a psychiatrist who specializes in brain neurochemistry. Again, the obligatory genetic analysis of George's blood detects no abnormalities; if it had, the subsequent therapy would have been tailored to normalize any aberrant neurotransmitter receptors. A prescription is written for "creatogogue," a synthetic neurotransmitter substance that will act to release a short burst of George's creativity. A completely safe substance, George can take the pill every day when he paints. Two years later, at George's first gallery showing, he turns down twenty-five thousand dollars for one of his favorite paintings and instead gives it to his psychiatrist.

Erin, a thirty-three-year-old mother of two-year-old twins, is having cabin fever. She has no real regrets about having at least temporarily given up her career as an assistant professor of archaeology, but in many ways longs for some stimulating human contact. So draining are her days caring for her babies, she has trouble remembering her exciting life before motherhood. It seems all she's ever done s change diapers, feed infants and set up mobiles. Of course she loves her children, but it would be wonderful to take a brief sojourn back to Florence, where she visited four years ago while examining the Etruscan ruins near Fiesole.

That afternoon she sees her opportunity and seizes it. While the twins mercifully nap, Erin dissolves the packet of powder she has gotten from her physician in some water, drinks it, closes her eyes and waits. Within five minutes she is transformed in her mind to the Viale Michaelangelo on an early autumn morning. The golden brown hue of the sunshine hitting the Forte Belvedere, the smell of baking bread wafting from the *panifici,* the well-dressed elderly Florentines out for a morning stroll, carrying their copies of *La Nazione,* and, of course, the famous panorama of the city below are so real they bring tears of joy to her eyes, the same way they did when she visited Firenze in the flesh. The journey takes only fifteen minutes clock time, and she awakes while her twins are still asleep, but the interlude makes Erin feel as if she just spent a week in Italy. For the first time in two years, Erin feels beautiful and elegant. Being able to "escape" every now and then will make her a much better mother.

Besides being a neurochemical factory, our brain is also a high-powered electrical plant. While the psychopharmacologists and molecular biologists are working to decipher and manipulate neurotransmitter receptor function, the biomedical engineers are working on the circuitry of our brain. The two disciplines merge beautifully in the area of memory enhancement. The processes by which we remember are more easily definable than the somewhat abstract self-esteem, creativity and imagination, and it is in this area that we will see the first applications of neuroscience to enhancing our daily lives.

In an experiment he conducted on Stanford University students in the 1970s, Dr. Kenneth Davis, now the chairman of the department of psychiatry at Mt. Sinai School of Medicine in New York, discovered that administering the drug physostigmine increased their ability to memorize a list of words by 10 to 20 percent. Physostigmine is an inhibitor of the enzyme in the brain that breaks down acetylcholine, a neurotransmitter involved in memory (and the one that is most decreased in the brains of patients with Alzheimer's disease). The Stanford students had no neurochemical deficiencies—on the contrary, they were all intelligent—so even a relatively small increase of memory in a group already performing close to optimal levels is remarkable, like a sub-four-minute miler taking two seconds off his best time.

And with the biochemical pathways responsible for memory being disentangled more every year, we're not too far away from the day when even more powerful memory-enhancing compounds will be available. The greatest results will be seen with those people who have the most room for improvement, but superior students will see gains, too, more even than in the early Stanford tests.

Memory is the area in which the biomedical engineers have already made significant advances. Using neural networking and artificial intelligence concepts, they are preparing to give the brain a high level of information processing ability, causing it to function as a high-speed computer. Before 2010, there will be an artificial brain that can manipulate numbers quickly, solve equations and learn whole banks of data—such as a new language—at once.

This new brain will find its first use in patients who have suffered premature memory loss—those with Alzheimer's disease or stroke—but shortly thereafter it will be used to reverse some of the signs of normal age-related memory loss. Finally, it will be used to improve memory in young, healthy people. The artificial device will not be a total brain substitute but the neurological equivalent of devices that are already in use called ventricular assist devices or VADs. These instruments don't replace all the functions of the heart, just the pumping of the left ventricle. Together with the new memory-boosting drugs that will be available, this new brain will allow us to learn and recall with blinding speed.

Ten years later, by 2020, this will be carried even further, with a genuine interface between the organic brain and a synthetic computer. Just as we now insert microchip-laden cards onto the mother boards of our computers, we will be able to have the same thing done to the brain, except the circuit cards will be constructed of both synthetic chips and fetal brain cells, which can be genetically engineered to cure disease. This is already being tested on Parkinson's disease, with the brain cells cultured by Dr. Snyder at Johns Hopkins, and it will be tested soon on Alzheimer's disease. Eventually it will be used to enhance normal brain function.

Euphoria drugs, drugs to enhance concentration, drugs to stimulate creativity, imagination powders, artificial brains. Aren't these just new names for hallucinogens, speed and cocaine, the counterculture of past decades gone mainstream? What kind of a society are we going to create?

A much better one. The brain biochemical or electrical modulators of 2020 will bear no resemblance in their effects to the LSD and mescaline of the sixties or seventies, or even to any legal drugs of today. Along with the application of computer circuitry, fetal nerve cell cultures and cloning techniques, with laserlike efficiency these compounds of the future will be able to turn up the speed and power on just one neurochemical reaction in the brain, without affecting others at all. Imagine how much better you could be at whatever you do if you could occasionally take something that would make you more confident, more creative, enhance your self-esteem. Imagine how it would improve business productivity.

We already regularly use a primitive example of what's to come. Judith Wurtman, a neurochemist at Massachusetts Institute of Technology, believes that caffeine improves creativity, and those of us who drink coffee know what that little boost in our spirits feels like. By 2020, that boost will be severalfold greater, more targeted at creativity and free of side effects.

These will not be artificial feelings. Motivational speakers constantly preach that in order to become successful at whatever we do we should emulate what successful people do, that we should "fake it till we make it." Ingesting something to biochemically jump-start this process is no more artificial, and will be much more effective, than giving ourselves a pep talk. Once we see what we're capable of, we won't need the outside help, and even if we did, it will be no different from any other form of preparation.

Could these new brain-altering drugs create a homogeneous society, where everyone is smart, happy and creative? Every one of us will have the potential to be smarter, happier and more creative, but only within the limits of our genetic possibilities. Both the floor and the ceiling of human achievement and experience will be raised higher, but there will be no less heterogeneity than there is today. A nonartist won't be turned into an artist, but a genetically programmed and environmentally trained artist will be a better one. Rather than disconnect us from our feelings, the brain drugs of the future will put us in closer touch with them and give clearer expression to them. Our feelings and emotions will no longer be obstacles to happiness and success, but catapults.

This entire approach will fall under the realm of what is going to be a major medical and health trend in the future—enhancement therapy. Doctors are going to spend at least as much time enhancing the lives of the well as they will treating the sick, of whom there will be many fewer. We already have some enhancement therapies—cosmetic surgery and sports medicine to name just two—but they are decidedly rudimentary when compared with what will be available within a few decades.

# 4

# The Hospital in Your Living Room

THE FOLLOWING SCENARIOS ARE NOT PROJECTIONS OF SOME dream. They are based on interviews I've had with Dr. Daniel Schneck of Virginia Polytechnic Institute, Dr. David Eddy of Duke University, Dr. Arthur Caplan of the University of Minnesota School of Medicine, Dr. George Lundberg, editor-in-chief of the *Journal of the American Medical Association,* and others. While some of the details may vary as the next dozen or more years unfold, the essential descriptions of the hospital in your living room are from the world of reality. This *is,* therefore, more or less, what we can expect. In fact, the first-generation model of the "smart toilet," which you will read about in the anecdote that follows, has already been introduced in Japan.

Ben is awakened out of a pleasant dream by his voice clock. "Good morning. The time is 0645. The date is April 27, 1998. The outdoor temperature is 57 degrees Fahrenheit, 13.9 degrees Celsius. Air quality excellent. Forecast is partly cloudy, winds calm, high temperature 72 Fahrenheit, 22.2 Celsius. All commuter trains running on schedule. Avoid outer expressway if driving."

Today is the first day of Ben's promotion to art director at his advertising firm, and he is excited about the possibilities for finally implementing some of his creative ideas. He goes into the bathroom, urinates and flushes.

Instead of going immediately down the drain, the urine spins in the ceramic commode, being rapidly analyzed by the electronic sensors. While he waits for the results, Ben slips his arm through a cuff attached to a panel on the tank and notices with satisfaction that the readout on the amber-on-black monitor confirms a blood pressure of 110 over 70 and a pulse of 54, readings he has maintained for one week. He then sits on the seat and has his weight and body fat measured and recorded. One hundred fifty-seven pounds and 14 percent body fat. Good. He resolves to make certain not to let his new career responsibilities interfere with his fitness.

By the time he has finished with these measurements, the reading of his urinalysis is displayed on the screen. Glucose—negative. Protein—negative. Bacteria—occasional, probably from skin contaminant, as yesterday. Please repeat after cleansing skin. White blood cells in urine—none. Red blood cells—occasional.

Although he is in a bit of a hurry this morning, Ben drinks two glasses of water and, after shaving and showering, dutifully repeats the urine test. The bacteria have disappeared. However, the red blood cells do not disappear on reanalysis. Ben is concerned.

Everything goes beautifully at work that day in his corner office with a view of the river. Five people working under him help him with the routine work he had to do alone for years. With the assistance of his new staff, Ben begins designing a campaign for their latest client.

But two or three times during the day, Ben's mind flashes back to the reading he got that morning. What could that mean, red blood cells in his urine? Ben is by no means a hypochondriac, but he is very health conscious and treats any abnormality as potentially serious. Why not? Why else does he have all this home-monitoring equipment if not to fine-tune his health?

As soon as he arrives home, Ben goes into the bathroom and urinates. The three minutes while the electronic sensors analyze the specimen seem interminable. Finally there is a screen display. No glucose, no protein, no white blood cells, occasional red blood cells. Damn!

Now Ben is convinced it isn't an artifact. He goes to the voice-activated computer station in his study and speaks into the microphone: "Give me the health options menu." The menu appears on the screen:

1. Do you want to communicate information to your physician or set up an appointment?

*Yes*
*No*

Ben is quite concerned so he responds yes and sets up an appointment for the following day.

2. Do you want to input data?

*Urine*
*Blood*
*Physical parameters*
*Other*

3. Do you want signs and symptoms analysis?

Ben instructs the computer that he wants option three.

"Please indicate the signs or symptoms, one at a time."

Ben speaks into the computer: "Red blood cells in the urine."
"How many?"
"Occasional."
"Are there any bacteria or white blood cells?"
"No."
"Is there any pain or fever?"
"No."
The optical disc whirs for fifteen seconds, after which a list of the most likely diagnoses appears on the screen.

1. Systemic lupus erythematosus
2. Tumor of kidney, bladder or urethra
3. Benign hematuria

If you would like more information about any of these, choose by number.
Ben chooses number three.

After just a few seconds, the screen fills: "In some people, blood appears in the urine for no apparent reason and is not associated with any disease. This is called benign hematuria and can be a hereditary condition or can be associated with intense physical activity. Have you a family history of blood in the urine or have you participated in any strenuous physical activity recently without adequate hydration?"

Ben answers yes and begins to feel a sense of relief. Just yesterday, he had gone for a sixteen-mile run with two of his friends, as they trained for their first triathlon coming up in three weeks. He knew that he hadn't drunk enough electrolyte replacement fluid during the run, and had been unusually thirsty for several hours afterward.

The computer tells Ben further that dehydration can cause minor trauma to the wall of the urinary bladder, which can cause painless bleeding in the urine, often visible only under a microscope. It should disappear within twenty-four hours, especially after adequate rehydration. If it does not, a physician appointment is suggested. The next morning when Ben checks his urine, there are no red blood cells.

Although he no longer needs to be concerned, Ben keeps the scheduled appointment anyway. He hasn't seen his doctor in several months and decides this is a good opportunity for an update. When he goes to the office, he is armed with a portfolio of personal medical information that he has been monitoring himself since his last visit. Ben gives his data to the nurse, and while he waits a few minutes in the waiting room, his physician studies the material. By keeping track of things that in the past his doctor would have had to do, Ben not only saves himself and his health insurance company thousands of dollars, but allows for the precious time with his physician to be used much more effectively. The thirty minutes they spend together are an intimate period of informed caring and an opportunity for fine-tuning his overall program. Ben leaves the office reassured and renewed.

In another household in 2005 Brett checks her computer for her daily schedule and is alerted by the blinking red highlight that it is time for her weekly blood tests for her entire family. She goes into the bathroom, opens the Plexiglas case and clips an earring onto her left ear. Before leaving for work, Brett reminds her husband Conrad to do the same and clips one to her young son's ear as well. In keeping with the fashion of the day, Brett's teenage daughter prefers a noseclip. Brett and Conrad go about their day, meet friends for dinner and, when they arrive home that evening, spend some time with their children. They all go to sleep and the next morning remove their clips. One at a time, they attach the earrings and nose ring with an adapter to their computer and via modem transmit the information about their blood tests to their physician's computer. Instead of using their computer software to interpret their results, they comply with their physician's request to transmit their analyses directly to his office to be monitored there and then be filed.

Amazingly, the entire process has taken place without drawing even a drop of blood. The earrings that Brett and her family wore are "functional jewelry." Attractively designed to be worn in public, these are highly sensitive analytical instruments. The ear and nose are good sites for the analysis because of the superficial blood capillaries present there. On the inside of the earrings and nose-clip—the part closest to the capillaries—are lasers that detect the molecular structure of every substance that flows past. There is also a resident computer chip that compares the structure of the compounds the lasers detect with a known map of all blood sub-stances programmed into the computer chip—such as cholesterol, including HDL and LDL and apolipoprotein fractions, glucose, sodium, potassium, antibody concentrations, vitamin levels, levels of drugs to monitor therapy, even early mutations in oncogenes (cancer-activating genes). Additional software in the chip allows for quantitative analysis of the substances detected.

Even though Brett and her family have been performing their analyses this way for three years now, since 2002, they are still in awe of the technology—although the effectiveness of home testing was fully established in the 1980s with the availability of fully automated monitors of blood pressure and glucose. The direct ac-cess laboratories that were so popular in the mid to late nineties, where people could walk in off the street to a licensed laboratory and order virtually any blood test they wanted, had been an im-provement over the old time-consuming, inconvenient and expen-sive practice of having to schedule an appointment with their physician, have the blood test and then go back for another ap-pointment for interpretation of the results. But they were light-years away in technology and ease compared with the way they are able to monitor their health now.

Their physician is impressed as well. Besides the obvious advantage to patients of a bloodless blood test, this method of analysis is more accurate than what was standard fifteen years earlier. Since almost every substance in our bodies is present in different concentrations at different times of the day, or even from day to day, one of the inherent problems of the older method of laboratory analysis was that it gave us a picture of only one moment in time, a snapshot. What is needed is an ongoing picture—a movie. That is what this family has now. Previously, patients may have been treated unnecessarily for elevated cholesterol while others with high cholesterol were not treated at all because judgments were based on one-time readings. The frequent and day-long monitoring of blood parameters in 2005 circumvents these possibilities. Using the laser clips, patients perform their own analyses on close to a weekly basis and electronically transmit the results either to their own or to the physician's computer. Each day the computer is instructed to quickly scan the laboratory parameters and, according to programmed instructions, alert the physician if any values have changed enough for concern.

The following day, Brett and Conrad receive a message on their home voice mail system from the physician's assistant at the Health Maintenance Organization they belong to: "Thank you for transmitting your latest blood tests. All of Brett's and the children's results are within optimal range and have deviated only an acceptable two percent since last week's reading.

"Conrad has had a fluctuation in his cholesterol. The LDL cholesterol and apolipoprotein B that carry the LDL have both risen eight percent since the last reading. In addition, the vitamin E level is down six percent. We have also noticed that Conrad has not transmitted blood results to us for an entire month. We are aware that he travels frequently on business. This procedure, however, can be done anywhere and the results either stored until arrival at home or transmitted to us through the internal modem in your laptop computer. Please be more diligent in the future. Test and transmit weekly if possible. Another reminder. Our mainframe computer indicates that the entire family needs to have yearly maintenance on their laser chips. This is essential in order to maintain accuracy in the analyses.

"We suggest that Conrad have an appointment to discuss fine-tuning his cellular biochemistry. Appointment times can be scheduled through your home computer link to our office. If a personal visit is not possible—and one is not required at this time—a fifteen-minute video appointment can be scheduled between 0600 and 2100 Monday through Friday. This can also be scheduled through your computer."

Conrad is leaving on a business trip for two weeks, so he schedules a video appointment three days hence from Los Angeles. By means of fiberoptic cables, a video image of his physician will be transmitted through the telephone onto large in-the-wall television screens that are a standard feature of most homes and hotels in the early twenty-first century. At the same time, Conrad's image will be transmitted to his physician, and through the telephone speaker they will be able to have a two-way conversation. Although it doesn't completely replace the personal contact necessary in some cases, it is a convenient and frequently used substitute for an in-office visit. Since the technology will already be in homes and hotels for other, nonmedical purposes, it adds nothing to the cost of medical care.

During the appointment, Conrad's physician reiterates that he needs to lower his LDL cholesterol and his apolipoprotein B by 8 percent and raise his vitamin E concentration by 6 percent in order to protect his LDL cholesterol from becoming oxidized and more likely to promote atherosclerosis. Since it had been determined five years earlier that constant monitoring and adjustment of tissue levels of many substances was beneficial in stopping disease in its molecular tracks, the doctor reminds Conrad that it is important to his future health for him to follow through on these recommendations. Weekly checking of several blood and tissue parameters has become integrated into the routines of most people's lives.

Conrad's values are not too far from what has been previously determined as optimal for him on his individual profile analysis, so medication will not be necessary. Instead, it is suggested that he visit the supermarket when he returns home to purchase a stock of "nutriceuticals," biotechnologically engineered foods that contain disease-fighting properties. In advance of that, he is directed to restaurants that serve nutriceutical meals in cities he will be visiting. Conrad's physician predicts that it should take approximately one month for his values to return to optimal levels but encourages him to perform an analysis and electronically transmit the results weekly to make certain that his profile is moving in the right direction. When the conversation is finished, Conrad's physician faxes directly to Conrad's hotel room a list of the recommended nutriceuticals he is to buy.

When Conrad telephones Brett later, he tells her about the conversation with his doctor and asks if she would mind shopping for him. Not at all, Brett says. She could handle all her supermarket purchases by accessing the store computer with her own, but she needs to go out anyway to get the laser chip for their blood analyzers serviced. Besides, it's a beautiful day and she wants the exercise. Body weight and composition are now easily controllable through specially designed foods, and even the endorphin release of aerobic exercise can be safely mimicked biochemically, but like many people, Brett often prefers the "natural" method.

Supermarkets in 2005 have become the health centers of the future, providing both products and education. Being able to custom-design diets for our particular health needs is just one of the services they provide. As nutrition has become more and more of a high-tech discipline, and nutriceuticals are peppered throughout every aisle of the store, the distinction between food and pharmacy has blurred. The in-store computers are able to quickly provide a complete nutritional analysis of any product on sale and even compare the relative nutritional merits of one product with another.

Supermarkets have also become environmentally conscious. Most foods are now genetically engineered to resist microorganisms, and packages themselves safely preserve food, eliminating the need for pesticides and preservatives.

But now let's get on with our story. Brett's seventy-three-year-old mother has recently been diagnosed as having insulin-dependent diabetes. It had been recognized for some time that a genetic predisposition to diabetes does exist, and the complex of genes was finally identified two years earlier, in 2003. Since that discovery, scientists have been hot on the trail of learning just how these abnormal genes cause diabetes, knowing that when the entire sequence was finally elucidated, there would be a whole host of new treatments. Until then, however, insulin continues to be the mainstay of therapy. But insulin therapy in 2005 is very different from what it had been in 1992. Brett takes her mother to her physician's office for the installation of a miniature artificial pancreas that will synchronize her insulin therapy precisely to her body's needs.

The artificial pancreas, the culmination of a major technological achievement which began to take shape in the early 1990s, is a semipermeable membrane into which have been inserted thousands of genetically engineered cells. These cells, grown in a laboratory, have been fitted with genes that allow them to mimic the action of the pancreas's beta cells which, when functioning properly, produce and secrete insulin and control blood sugar.

Remarkably, the artificial pancreas doesn't have to be surgically placed in the abdomen where the pancreas is normally located. The physician's assistant makes a small incision and implants the tiny device under the skin on the underside of the left arm. It is now able to sense exactly what the blood sugar concentration is at all times and secrete the precise dose of insulin needed to keep the sugar under control.

There will never again be a need for Brett's mother to prick her finger and check her blood sugar or to have to inject herself with insulin every day. It is all being done automatically, a method not only much more convenient, but far more precise and one that will markedly reduce diabetic complications.

Now it is autumn, 1999, and we meet Glynn, who has received a letter from the National Health Information Service, asking her to participate in an upcoming patient focus group. Glynn recalls vividly what health care used to be like. In the early nineties, the United States was spending 12 percent of its gross national product—$600 billion—on health care, and by 1995 it went up to almost $800 billion. Everyone was talking about the runaway train of health care inflation. And despite all this money spent, there were almost forty million Americans without any health insurance, and another fifty million who were underinsured. She remembers watching a television symposium about possible solutions during which the only one who made any sense to her was a Dr. David Eddy from Duke University, who said that, as in any other service in the marketplace, the consumer has to be involved in how much is spent. After all, he said, the costs of health care are passed on to patients, in the form of either reduced benefits or higher taxes. By 1996, the government began to listen and implement Dr. Eddy's plan.

In June, 1996, Glynn and her husband had each received a plastic "smart card" in the mail, with a booklet of instructions on how it was to be used. Glynn would carry it with her to every "health encounter" she would have—whether it was a visit to her doctor, a trip to the pharmacy to fill a prescription, to a clinic, to a hospital.

When presented, the smart card will be passed over an ultraviolet sensor to identify her, just as when she pays a bill at a restaurant with a credit card. Her entire health history is now available at a glance and more data will be added as a result of this visit. All the information on Glynn is in a huge national data bank called the National Health Informatin System. Privacy is a concept belonging to the past.

As new information is collected on Glynn, it will be analyzed by experts. If Glynn were a candidate for coronary angioplasty, the data would be studied by cardiovascular surgeons; if she were a child with measles, pediatricians would do the analyzing. Other authorities would then scrutinize the costs, benefits and dangers of all the procedures. This same information will then be available to activist patient groups throughout the country, going into a data bank that will be used as a basis for formulating universal low-cost health insurance.

Now for another scenario: In 2012, a family celebrates the fourth birthday of their child, silently giving thanks for her perfect health. This has not been a matter of luck, but of design, even though their child has never been inside a hospital and has been to the doctor only once in her four years.

Their daughter, born at home in 2008, was delivered by her father. Until the late 1990s all home births were performed by either obstetricians or midwives. But by 2005, a growing number of fathers were expressing a desire to be even more active participants in the birth of their children. Parent deliveries became commonplace by 2008—as a high-tech process that would not have been familiar to a twentieth-century midwife.

As long as the delivery was going to be an uncomplicated one—and this could be predicted well in advance—the delivery technique would be easy to teach to prospective fathers and would be included in standard prenatal instruction classes. It would go something like this. When your wife begins labor, attach to her abdomen the sensing electrode which will continually check the heartbeat, blood pressure, and respiration of both mother and baby as well as measure the force of the mother's uterine contractions. The other end of the electrode should then be hooked to the modem on your telephone that transmits information through a fiberoptic cable to your doctor's office. Not only will vital signs be visible on a monitor but the obstetrician will view the entire delivery procedure on a television screen. By speakerphone, father and physician will communicate throughout the entire birth. During parental classes the father will have been trained in emergency procedures. But thanks to advanced prenatal monitoring, emergency intervention is needed in fewer than one in five thousand home births.

Following the easy birth, the father attaches to the baby's scalp a miniature version of the laser clips the parents regularly use to perform blood analyses on themselves. This tests the baby for the inherited disease phenylketonuria, or PKU, as well as all the other genetic abnormalities that can be tested for in 2008. The results are transmitted to their pediatrician via modem.

For the first week, the baby sleeps with both of her parents, intensifying the bonding process. By the second week, though, it is time for her to sleep in her crib. In the past, this had always been a time of some concern for parents. Sudden infant death syndrome (SIDS), or "crib death," was an uncommon occurrence but statistics of its rarity were never reassuring. In 2008, there is less to worry about, since the baby's crib is equipped with a monitoring system previously available only in the neonatal intensive care units of hospitals.

Embedded in the mattress is a group of sensors able to detect any abnormalities in respiration, pulse, blood pressure, oxygen content of the blood or any seizurelike activity of the leg muscles (so-called myoclonus, an early sign of SIDS). If any of these occurred, a computer would automatically activate a pulmonary stimulation device that would improve the baby's breathing, increase the oxygen content of the air and simultaneously sound an alarm in the parents' bedroom. The crisis alleviated, the parents could alert their pediatrician, who would test the child further the next day. Fortunately, none of this happened with this baby.

As with any new technology, when first introduced in 2005, the monitoring system was expensive—more than five thousand dollars—and was optional equipment on cribs, although it was considered a medical expense and as such was tax deductible. Within just a few years, though, many manufacturers were offering the equipment, bringing the cost down to less than one third the original price, and the monitoring system became standard equipment.

In addition, the baby's room is equipped with instruments to electronically measure and record her height and weight, so there is no need for the six-week well-baby checkup with the pediatrician. At three months old, the baby is taken for her first and only visit to her doctor. All the information on the child has been regularly transmitted by the parents, so the physical exam is only a brief confirmation of what had already been determined by the in-home monitoring equipment, that this is a perfectly healthy baby. The physician has time for a relaxed visit with the family.

Before the parents leave, the pediatrician gives them eight color-coded capsules to be put sequentially in the baby's food starting the following month and continuing for seven more months. Each of the capsules contains genetically engineered vaccines and altogether will protect against all the childhood diseases. The active principles in the viruses were identified years ago, and it thus became possible to design safer and more effective vaccines, as well as coating them to protect them from the action of the protein-dissolving stomach and intestinal enzymes. This enabled all the vaccines to be given orally.

Newborn infants are not the only ones who will need to be closely monitored for health problems. Those at the other end of the spectrum—older people—are even more vulnerable. They will not be neglected by the technology of the future. The medical paging devices that are available today are beneficial, but they are only a prelude to what's coming. Instead of having to rely on someone who may be too sick, or even unconscious, to press a button and call for help, the rescue process will be initiated automatically. Nothing will be left to chance.

The monitors that we will wear will not look much different from the ubiquitous plastic watches of today. But in addition to telling the time and being an athletic performance aid, they will be sophisticated monitors that continually watch over our heart rate, blood pressure, brain waves and respiration. Anytime there is a significant deviation from what has been programmed into the software as normal, a radio signal will alert our doctor, who will wear a chronometer as a receiver.

Further down the road—we're calling for it to appear at about 2020—our ability to handle medical problems in our homes will reach a level of sophistication that most of us wouldn't even dream possible today. Not only will we have the capability of diagnosing diseases, but we will be able to effectively treat them without seeing a physician.

Imagine the following in 2020: a healthy thirty-six-year-old woman notices that it is time for her monthly checkup. As most people do, she follows the practice of regularly testing her blood and transmitting the results to her physician, but not everything can be detected by blood analysis. She needs to check her entire body for evidence of any early abnormalities.

Impregnated right into her showerhead is an optical computer scanner, with a small screen attached. Most days the unit remains off but today she activates the scan mode and her entire body is silently and deeply probed, right down to the cellular level, while she takes her shower. When she has finished, and while she dresses, the computer in the scanning unit begins analyzing the results. There is no reason to expect anything different, since she has always been in perfect health, but the computer is taking longer this month. The screen displays the message: "One moment please. Analyzing data."

After another two minutes a diagram appears on the screen, with the following message. "Scanning has revealed a three-micron area of cells with atypical metabolism in the upper outer quadrant of the left breast as depicted on the accompanying diagram." She notices a tiny highlighted area in her left breast. "There are no malignant cells, but if left untreated there is a one in thirty chance that within three years there will be malignant changes. Advise eliminating this cluster of cells immediately. For your pharmacist, the code number for this lesion is 36-A."

Although the woman is horrified that she actually has some abnormal cells growing inside her, the same thing has happened to one of her friends and she knows her friend was able to take care of the problem easily, so she remains calm. She immediately telephones her pharmacist, gives him the code number, and he promises to have the necessary medication delivered to her within an hour.

The delivery from the pharmacy is a small bottle that contains only one tiny pinkish white capsule that resembles the vitamins she takes every morning. Could this actually be the treatment for her breast abnormality? The woman swallows the capsule, somehow expecting to feel something unleashed from this powerful medication, but after several hours feels nothing.

Three days later, she repeats the scan as the computer had recommended. This time, the scanner finds no abnormality: "The atypical cells located on previous scan have been eradicated. Please repeat scan next month according to regular schedule."

The capsule that the woman swallowed contained a genetically engineered monoclonal antibody to the particular kind of atypical cells in her breast, identified by the code number the computer generated. Attached to the monoclonal antibody was a cellular toxin. Once the antibody homed in on the abnormal cells—and only the abnormal cells—the toxin entered the cells and destroyed them before the tumor could gain a foothold. The focus of abnormal cells was so submicroscopic (three ten-thousandths of a centimeter) that even sensitive mammography wouldn't have been able to detect it for at least another two years.

The advances that are going to make this home medical care possible are going to be truly amazing, but no more so than what we have witnessed in the past twenty-five years. Would you have believed it in 1965 if someone had told you that in 1992 your ten-year-old child would be able to program a computer, or that there would be machines that would be able to look inside your body without x-rays and in far greater detail? Twenty years from now, we will have discovered different energy patterns emitted by the body that will make the CAT scans and MRI imaging of today outmoded. And the new technology will be cheap, portable and available to all in their homes.

Is the ability to diagnose and treat most diseases in our homes going to put our doctors out of work? Not at all. On the contrary, there are going to be so many breakthroughs in so many complex areas that if we weren't able to manage most of our health problems by ourselves, our doctors would be inundated and unable to provide any type of quality care at all. We're going to be able to free them up and then turn our contact with them into more intimate, productive sessions. Technology will actually bring us closer together.

# 5

# The Timing of Our Lives

OVER THE PAST TEN YEARS OR SO, LIKE A CREW OF GOOD WATCH-makers, chronobiologists—combining the disciplines of medicine, biology, physics, psychology and mathematics—have been intensely studying what it is that makes our biological clocks tick.

What they have discovered is that there is another dimension to our physiology just as important as the thousands of complex biochemical reactions that continually take place in our cells. Virtually every function in our body is on a timer—how alert we are, how well our blood clots, when our cells divide, how well we digest, how well we remember things, how strong we are. And all of these functions vary at a different rate—some change from minute to minute, others fluctuate by the hour, while still others oscillate on a daily, weekly, monthly or even yearly pattern.

We are a society accustomed to constancy, but since practically everything in our body works in wavelike rhythms rather than on a straight line, we now are beginning to recognize that constancy is not the best policy. In the next couple of decades, we're going to be paying serious attention to our biological clocks, adjusting to them when appropriate, but at other times resetting them. Either way, the impact on how almost every disease is diagnosed, treated and even prevented is going to be monumental. *When* something is done is going to assume as much significance as *what* it is that we are doing.

Human beings are not unique in the way they are affected by rhythms; in fact, rhythms are inherent to every living thing, plant or animal. This has been known for centuries, but it was only twenty years ago that the site of the biological clock (or, as chronobiologists usually call it, our circadian pacemaker) was identified. It is made up of two structures: one, just behind the eyes, a cluster of cells from the hypothalamus (part of the brain) called the suprachiasmatic nucleus (SCN), the other the pineal gland, just a few centimeters away. Seventeenth-century French philosopher and mathematician René Descartes thought the pineal gland was the seat of the soul. While later scientists dismissed that notion, until the pineal was found to be an integral part of our body timer, no other function for it was discovered. It was thought to be like our appendix, a vestigial structure. But now we know otherwise.

The pineal gland and the SCN operate together to cue the rest of our body, sending hormonal messages through the bloodstream or electronic signals through the nervous system. It is through this communication that the daily, weekly, monthly or yearly variations in function occur.

It is no accident of nature that the biological clock is so closely related to the eye. The light-dark cycle is one of the primary stimuli of our body timer. The most obvious example of this is sleep. Darkness hitting the SCN sends a message to the pineal gland to begin pouring a hormone called melatonin, a sleep-inducing substance, into the bloodstream. Bright light hitting the SCN turns off melatonin production. In somewhat more complex ways, the same light-dark cycles, along with weaker cues such as mealtime and periods of activity, also send signals throughout our body to subsidiary biological clocks that control every cell process.

Chronobiologists have also found that, while the basic mechanism is the same, the functioning of our biological clocks differs from person to person, inherited in our genes. Some work better at different times and some just don't work very well at all. This can both make us much less than optimally productive and increase our risk for disease. Better understanding of the precise mechanisms by which the biological clocks signal all of our metabolism, as well as learning more about the genes that control the individual differences, is going to help all our biological clocks run as smoothly as a Rolex within the next ten years.

Let's look at David, a frequent traveler from New York to Tokyo, and project him just a bit into the future, to 1998. When his secretary makes his reservation through the in-office computer, instructions appear on the screen that if he plans to be active immediately upon arrival in Japan, David should exercise that morning and eat a light breakfast. He boards his flight in midafternoon, to find that dinner is served within thirty minutes of takeoff. Two hours later, an announcement is made that the cabin is going to be darkened, and although there are intense quartz halogen lamps for reading and individual monitors for watching a movie without disturbing fellow passengers, sleep is recommended in order to avoid jet lag upon arrival.

The delicious meal (an innovation in itself), the cabin's darkness, the comfortable and ample reclining seats and the soothing music pumped through his headphones cause David to drift asleep even though it is only six o'clock in the evening in New York. After six and one-half hours of rest, the stewardess gently awakens him. She informs him that there are approximately four hours till landing in Narida Airport and that he should use the light goggles she is distributing. David puts on the plastic opaque goggles and flicks the switch on the side. He is immediately enveloped in bright fluorescent light that delivers a measured dose directly to the retina, from where it is transferred to the SCN, his biological clock. This amount of light sends a clear message to the clock: time to get up and be alert; it is the beginning of a new day.

After just fifteen minutes with the light goggles, David feels as charged as if he had just slept eight hours in his own bed and had his usual huge mug of morning coffee. In order to feel in the flow of a normal day, David now has breakfast, but he doesn't need the stimulation of caffeine. He takes his laptop out of his briefcase and, just as he does every morning on his commute into New York, works for two hours. He further organizes on the bullet train to Osaka and delivers the business presentation of his life. When he arrives back home four days later (reversing the process) David feels both exhilarated and rested, two foreign feelings after an international trip.

• • •

With some variation, we will use these methods to adopt to all travel across more than two time zones. How and when we use the sleep-wake cycles will depend on which direction we are flying. Another accommodation the airlines will make by 1998 is to schedule flights that synchronize better with our biological clocks.

For example, consider the flight from New York to London, an especially difficult one, as anyone who has flown it can attest to. It's not that long—only about two hours longer than a flight from New York to Los Angeles—but there are two differences that make it more strenuous. First, the flight to LA crosses only two time zones whereas the London flight crosses five time zones. Second, and more important, most flights from New York to London depart in the evening and arrive in London at six o'clock in the morning London time, but it's only one in the morning New York time. The wee hours of the morning are the time when our biological clocks are most vulnerable to being upset by bright light. Exposing them on arrival in London—which the airlines do to us even before landing by opening the shades, turning on the cabin light and feeding us breakfast, trying to pretend that we've had a good night's sleep on the relatively short hop, just when our body is telling us it's ready to go to sleep—shoots our biological clocks more westward toward Hawaii, making it even more difficult for us to adapt.

Chronobiologists, including Dr. Martin Moore-Ede, director of the Institute for Circadian Physiology in Boston, are working with the airlines. When we met in his office he told me of two solutions that will occur by 1998. First, there will be hotels right in the airport terminals, holding places after arrival that will be included in the price of the ticket. Upon arrival in London or Paris or Zurich or any other European city in the same time zone, we will be whisked into comfortable rooms for a three-hour nap, while representatives of the airlines check our bags through customs. Then, we will be awakened and given a fifteen-minute dose of the fluorescent-light goggles. Just this three-hour rest period will put us at New York time of four in the morning, a time when our biological clocks are easily set toward Europe rather than Hawaii. It will only be a little after nine in the morning in Europe, but we will feel as if we've had a good night's sleep.

The other solution is that more and more airlines will begin offering flights that leave the United States in the morning and arrive at early evening in Europe. Since it will be early afternoon U.S. time, we will be wide awake. We'll go out, have a wonderful late night in London or Paris, go to sleep and allow our biological clocks to slip into synch with the new time.

Further in the future, by about 2005, there will be easier and better ways to reset our biological clocks. As travel speeds increase, and we routinely cross more and more time zones, being able to do this will assume even greater importance. Instead of using light and appropriately timed rest periods, we will simply take an anti-jeg-lag pill, not the nostrums that are available over the counter today but remedies based on solid science. At first, according to Dr. Josephine Arendt, a chronobiologist at the University of Surrey in England, we will take a capsule of melatonin, the pineal gland hormone involved in the sleep-wake cycle. She has published several papers demonstrating that there are no side effects of melatonin and that it effectively resets our biological clocks to new time zones. Dr. Arendt has already begun testing the effects of melatonin pills on men in Britain's research base in Antarctica, where the sun essentially disappears for three months during the southern hemisphere winter, severely disrupting circadian pacemakers. Soon this research will be applied to the rest of us.

But scientists are beginning to discover that melatonin is not the only hormone involved in our biological clocks. A group of neuroscientists at Georgia State University, led by H. Elliot Albers, have identified at least three additional substances that help regulate the sleep-wake cycle, all of them neurotransmitters, the chemical messengers in our brain. Two of these neurotransmitters are more active at night, the other during the day, and Dr. Albers found that injecting one or more of these into a rat alters the biological clock to whatever time was desired. These findings are early, but within about ten years, we will see application of them to ease jet lag.

While jet lag is something nearly all of us have experienced, since it occurs infrequently, it poses no danger to our health. There are conditions, though, in which the disruption of our biological clock occurs more frequently, and in these cases there is an increased risk for disease.

About twenty-one million people in the United States alone work on shifts, rotating from days (7 to 3) to nights (11 to 7) to evenings (3 to 11), usually at weekly intervals. "It is like spending a week in Denver, a week in Paris and a week in Tokyo," says Dr. Moore-Ede, "perpetual jet lag." Not unexpectedly, these people perform more poorly on their jobs than those who have regular hours. Shift workers don't just include the clerk in the all-night supermarket, but those on whom our society depends for optimal performance: policemen, petrochemical workers, the nuclear power industry, the airlines, truckers and—ironically—health care workers. The Three-Mile Island, Chernobyl and Bhopal disasters all took place at night, more likely due to an upsetting of biological clocks than coincidence.

And there are consequences to the workers as well. Even those who work permanent night shifts never adapt well. Despite their diminished alertness on the job, many of them suffer from daytime insomnia, unable to sleep during daylight hours while the rest of the world goes about their business. Because of these disruptions to their timers, they are far more prone to heart attacks, ulcers, problems with reproduction (especially in women) and depression.

Until recently, most industries arranged their schedules solely to maximize economic output, without taking into account the biological time clocks of their workers. Whether it has been motivated by fears of liability over poor performance or concern for the health of the workers, attention is now being paid to circadian rhythms in those who must work at night.

What is becoming standard is switching the rotation of shifts to a clockwise one (day-evening-night) rather than the more common counterclockwise one (day-night-evening). Chronobiologists have advised that this is more in tune with our biological clocks and adaptation is 50 percent easier. But a more effective method will soon be in place in most industries. It focuses on the use of the same type of bright lights that will help alleviate jet lag.

Dr. Charles Czeisler of Harvard Medical School has already shown that this works. He instructed night-shift workers to remain in the dark from nine in the morning to five in the afternoon (their windows were covered with opaque material to exclude sunlight) and exposed them to bright light, equivalent to sunlight, throughout their entire shift. Within just one week, most of their biological clocks perfectly adapted, evidenced by normal body temperature and secretion of hormones, both of which are abnormal in shift workers whose biological clocks have not adapted. And, equally as important, their mental functions and performance were superior to a control group whose light-dark cycle wasn't adjusted. As a result of this demonstrated adaptability, shift changes will be at longer intervals (e.g., monthly) to accommodate the physiology of the workers.

Within five years, specially constructed bright lights that deliver a measured dose of sunlight-equivalent will become a standard fixture in hospitals, nuclear power plants and airline cockpits. Those more mobile—such as truck drivers and policemen—will be required to wear on duty mini-versions of what will be in institutions, special bright-light-delivering goggles similar to those that will help alleviate jet lag (but which will deliver the light in such a way that it directly hits the retina without interfering with vision). Because they will be as alert as a day worker, their performance will dramatically improve. We will all be better off for it, and the incidence of health complications in the workers will markedly decrease.

What will also be discovered with further research is that not everyone's biological clock adapts equally well, the consequence of genetics. We've all seen examples of this. Some of us are "morning people," others are "night people," and our biological clocks tell us which part of the day to gravitate toward to do our best work. Some of us are more affected by jet lag than others. My next-door neighbor is an internationally acclaimed photographer and is constantly flying all over the world for *National Geographic* magazine. But he can take an eighteen-hour flight from Tibet and call us to go out to dinner the next night, whereas it takes me at least two or three days to feel normal after a trip to Los Angeles.

These individual differences in our biological clocks often persist despite intervention. Not all night-shift workers respond equally well to appropriately timed light therapy. By 1998, before anyone is hired for a position in which he will have to work at least part of the time at night, he will be tested to see if he can do so without adverse effects on either his performance or his health. Such applicants will be put through several days of job simulation, treated with the same light therapy they would be given if they actually get the job, and their adaptability will be gauged in a variety of ways—hormonal secretion, body temperature, sleep patterns, mental function. If they don't measure up to an objective standard, they will be termed "chronobiologically unemployable"—i.e., unemployable for shift work.

This will not be the same thing as "genetically unemployable"— something else we are going to have to deal with in the future, but which we will emphatically reject. The deplorable practice of refusing to hire people, not because they have a disease, but because they have merely inherited a predisposition is a discrimination that has no scientific merit. On the other hand, although our biological clocks are inherited, in the "chronobiologically unemployable," the poorly adaptable circadian timekeeper will not be a predisposition but will have already manifested itself. Because employing these people would be a detriment to both society and themselves, it will be more analogous to the eminently logical position of an airline refusing to hire a pilot who already has signs of heart disease.

This practice, though, will not have to last long. By about 2005, the same hormonal and neurochemical treatments that will be applied to ease jet lag will be used to help shift workers adapt their biological clocks. As these reactions are further teased apart into their separate phases, not only will employment testing become easier and more sophisticated—it will only involve measuring the levels of a variety of neurotransmitters—but it will be possible to adjust even the most genetically recalcitrant biological clock to the desired schedule. The ranks of the "chronobiologically unemployable" will be forever depleted.

Poorly running biological clocks are not just a problem for those who must work rotating shifts. There is solid evidence developing that the same malfunctioning is responsible for many cases of depression. Also by 1998, the diagnostic procedures used to detect abnormal circadian timers in shift workers, and the subsequent use of light and neurohormonal therapy, will find its way into psychiatrists' offices as standard care for many patients. In addition, the sleep problems many older people experience—those that aren't related to an accompanying depression—are not because we need less sleep when we get older. That is a fallacy. Rather, in several cases it is being demonstrated to be a disruption, or an aging, of their biological timekeeper. Instead of giving these people sleeping pills, by 1998 physicians will be giving them light goggles and by 2005 melatonin and neurotransmitter supplements.

The fire in northeast San Diego County was raging out of control for the fourth straight day. Thousands of acres had already been lost, at least that many animals had perished, and the fire was coming close enough to Alpine that they might have to evacuate the entire mountain town. The computers that were standard for forest fire fighters in 2012 were effectively projecting how rapidly the fire would burn and where the high-tech digging equipment should put the trenches and control lines, but this was one of the worst fires in years. The Santa Ana winds were roaring at fifty miles per hour and fanning the woods, burning like a charcoal grill at a cookout. The weather service had said that if the fire could be contained for another four days, the winds should die down and they would be able to finally bring the fire under control.

These were twenty-four-hour days, though. The fire didn't take breaks, and neither could the fire fighters. There were several of them on site, but almost all of them were needed all the time, and if they weren't at their sharpest mentally and physically, it could lead to disaster.

Although so many things were going against them, every crew member was functioning at one hundred percent of his capacity. The stainless steel trailer that had been set up for the fire fighters not only provided a place to eat and periodically clean up, but until recently something unheard of in the annals of emergency fire fighting: a place to sleep.

In the trailer was a computer programmed for a specific pattern. Each of the fifteen fire fighters was put on a schedule that required sleep for fifteen minutes at four-hour intervals around the clock. These intervals were not selected at random but carefully designed to correspond to the several periods during the day when the biological clocks of the fire fighters were most naturally "drowsy." When this system was first tried in 2007, fire fighters had been skeptical, just another scientific theory that wouldn't work. Although they were assured by the chronobiologists who had designed the program that it had been laboratory-tested for several years, the fire fighters assumed that six periods of fifteen minutes' sleep—only ninety minutes out of every twenty-four hours—was going to be worse than toughing it out and just staying awake straight through for several days. Yes, there had been some poor, even fatal, decisions made following the old pattern, but the thought of hitting the bed for fifteen minutes and having to immediately get up again seemed too disorienting to cope with.

But on instructions from their superiors, they agreed to try. The computer in their wristwatches was synchronized with the main computer in the trailer. If they were out fighting the fire and it came time for their sleep, the alarm on their watch would sound. Then, after fifteen minutes' sleep in the trailer, the alarm would sound again.

The results were amazing. Even though they each got only ninety minutes' sleep for as long as seventeen straight days, not one error in judgment was made because of mental or physical fatigue, and all of their vital signs being monitored stayed perfectly within optimal range. It became the standard operating procedure for emergency fire fighting.

The system implemented by the fire fighters is called polyphasic sleep. We've all heard stories that Leonardo da Vinci and Thomas Edison discovered that they could get by on as little as an hour and a half of sleep a day. And during the Cold War, from time to time there were mysterious reports from the Soviet Union that their engineers and scientists had developed a program for being productive on just a few hours' sleep a night. Whether this was scientific fact or propaganda was never documented. It wasn't until the 1990s that this began to be studied seriously and openly at the Institute for Circadian Physiology in Boston, the same laboratory where other experiments on the biological clock were being conducted.

The researchers found that polyphasic sleep did indeed work, if it was carefully controlled. The short naps must coincide exactly with the several periods during the day when our biological timekeepers are telling us to rest. Most of us experience this regularly but ignore it and keep on working. By following fluctuations in hormonal secretion and other physiological parameters, the scientists in Boston precisely identified these periods most amenable to rest (they occur approximately every four hours) and scheduled the sleep for those times.

In addition, because it sleeps so little, the body becomes ravenous for REM (rapid eye movement) sleep and reaches it almost instantly. REM is the deep sleep that we require in order to dream, feel rested and be at our mental and physical best. Under a more typical sleep pattern, it usually takes us more than one hour before we begin REM sleep.

Although properly controlled polyphasic sleep is not detrimental to our health at all, it still requires such a high degree of motivation that it won't be routinely adopted. But by working with our biological clocks this way, many other situations besides those of fire fighters will be improved. Space stations are going to become a definite fixture in our future, and there will often be instances in which those operating the space stations will be called upon to stay awake and alert for long periods at a time. Polyphasic sleep will be ideal for them. Even sooner, polyphasic sleep is going to be adapted to improve the medical profession. There have been several highly publicized cases in recent years of patients dying in hospitals because the medical resident made a fatal error in judgment. In light of the hours physicians-in-training are asked to keep, it is actually surprising that more of these disasters haven't occurred. One case in a prominent New York hospital led to a barrage of letters to medical journals calling for a revision of schedules for medical residents.

The schedules will be revised, but not by shortening hours, as has been called for. Physicians need to be present in long stretches not only to provide enough treatment for patients but so that they can be exposed during their residency to as many situations as possible. By 1997, instead of asking these young doctors to perform superhuman feats of stamina at the expense of patients, for their entire internship and residency they will adhere to a polyphasic pattern of sleep.

It is 1997 in the pathology department of a major medical center. A pathologist and a surgeon sit on opposite sides of a powerful two-headed microscope, examining a slide of the biopsy material of the lymph node the surgeon removed yesterday from the groin of his forty-six-year-old patient. The pathologist points out the numerous mitotic figures, the bizarre cell formations and the almost complete absence of any tissue organization, all evidence of how malignant the tumor is. In order for the patient to survive the cancer, chemotherapy will have to be started immediately.

The surgeon consults with the oncology department and his patient is transferred there that day. After a few preliminary tests, the chemotherapy is begun. But the chemotherapy that is begun in 1997 is substantially different from what has been used in the past. The drug itself is a new antitumor agent, a powerful one that oncologists have wanted to use for some time, but haven't been able to because it had proven too toxic to normal tissues. Under the innovative delivery systems now routinely used for chemotherapy, it is finally possible to use this potent agent.

Under local anesthesia, a large polyethylene capsule that resembles a syringe is implanted beneath the skin near the patient's waist, an area where subcutaneous tissue is reasonably thick. The capsule houses three drugs, the new powerful one and two others that have been proven effective against this type of poorly differentiated lymphoma. But besides containing the drugs, the capsule is also an implantable drug delivery system that is equipped with a biosensor and a computer.

Because of this unique device, the patient does not have to come to the hospital for his dose of chemotherapy. The drugs will be automatically administered several times each day. Since the trigger for their release will be the patient's own biological clock, they will be more effective and will not cause the devastating side effects that cancer patients have come to fear almost as much as having the disease itself.

The drug delivery system works like this. Each of the three drugs in the implanted syringe damages the cancer cells at different stages. One affects the cell's ability to take in nutrients; another inhibits DNA synthesis; and still another blocks cell division. Normal cells exhibit these same activities, but often not at the same time as the cancer cells. The goal for the most effective therapy with the fewest side effects is to administer each drug not only when it will be most effective against the cancer cells, but when it will be least damaging to normal cells.

Chemotherapy in 1992 pays little attention to this. The drugs are administered according to a predetermined, regular schedule, which kills some cancer cells (but not as many as could be killed) but also kills many normal cells—many more than should be killed.

But, by 1997, the research of chronobiologists will revolutionize chemotherapy. They have found that all of these cellular activities occur in rhythms, which are under the control of the body's biological clock. Each cell activity releases different biochemical byproducts into the circulation, and the products of cancer cells differ from those of normal cells. The sensors in the implantable syringe are programmed to detect not only whether the chemical signal is from a cancer cell or a normal cell, but also what the specific signal is. Depending on the signal, the sensor in turn sends a message to the attached computer to deliver a measured dose of the particular drug that responds to that signal. This system continually monitors cell activity so chemotherapy is automatically administered in accordance with the patient's biological clock, when it will be most effective against the cancer cells and least damaging to the normal tissue, making for a far better result.

Working with our biological timekeeper is going to change not only chemotherapy but a variety of other treatments, including some additional ones for cancer. In a later chapter, we are going to discuss several innovative treatments for cancer, many of which will be also administered in accordance with our biological clocks. And although surgery for cancer is eventually going to be outmoded, until that time it will be scheduled, in many cases, according to our biological clocks. As an example of the effectiveness of this approach, Dr. William Hrushesky of Albany Medical College told me that, because of the biological clock's influence on hormonal secretions, women operated on for breast cancer in midmenstrual cycle have a four times better chance of surviving than those operated on at either the beginning or the end of their cycles.

Surgery for other diseases, when it can be elective, will be dependent on our biological clocks too. There are a whole constellation of factors that determine how well we heal after surgery, and every one of them works in a rhythm. By 1998, before surgery is scheduled on any patient, the pattern of secretion of a variety of metabolic factors involved in tissue healing—growth factors, hormones, electrolytes, vitamins—will be determined so that the surgery can be timed for optimal recovery.

Besides the treatment of disease, chronobiology will play an important role in both the diagnosis and the prevention of disease. For many years, cardiologists have been applying this principle with the Holter monitor, the device that patients wear to record heart rhythms over a twenty-four-hour period, and the ambulatory blood pressure recorder. This will soon be extended to the diagnosis of almost all conditions. Just as surgery for breast cancer is most effective at a certain time of month, so is the diagnosis if a woman has a mammogram in accordance with her biological clock. The timing of Pap smears with a rhythmic pattern is important, and so too for many male cancer tests. When men schedule their prostate exams will depend on certain monthly or yearly fluctuations in hormones. Virtually every blood component is on a timer, and this will be taken into account when diagnostic blood tests are performed.

Diseases can be prevented by paying attention to how our biological clocks cause metabolic variations. Newborn infants from families with a history of high blood pressure show bigger daily swings in blood pressure than newborns from families without a history of hypertension. Within five years, the blood pressure of all newborn infants will be monitored with computers and sensors for the first forty-eight hours after birth to determine susceptibility to hypertension. This will enable us to begin preventive measures at the earliest possible time. Once the series of predisposing genes to hypertension is identified (between 2005 and 2010), neonatal monitoring will be limited to those babies.

By monitoring seasonal changes of the hormone prolactin in women with fibrocystic disease of the breast, chronobiologists have shown that it is possible to predict which of them will progress to breast cancer. The same can be done with continual temperature monitoring. Looking at biological rhythms such as these, and many more, will soon become a common way of identifying vulnerability to a disease at the earliest possible time, when intervention can abolish the pathology. Using sensors and computers, the analysis of these rhythms will become far more sophisticated and meaningful.

# PART II

# TIMELINE
# 1992-2030

*CURES TO EXPECT . . . AND WHEN*

*PROCEDURES THAT WILL CHANGE . . . AND WHY*

*PROBLEMS YOU CAN PREVENT . . . AND HOW*

THE FOLLOWING TIMELINE, AS PRECISELY AS POSSIBLE, CHARTS the development and the availability of a wide range of cures as well as diagnostic procedures and preventive techniques. This section provides a shorthand overview of medical progress which, for the most part, is discussed in greater detail elsewhere. Occasionally, though, you will find entries that are not expanded upon in other chapters. Those entries are somewhat longer and should satisfy the immediate concerns of most readers.

All predictions, no matter how well informed, are arbitrary in the sense that they very much depend on the bias of the predictor. Researchers tend to be conservative and so do I. Therefore, it is conceivable that some of these breakthroughs will occur somewhat earlier than I have predicted. This is more likely the further out we get in time. It is also possible that some of the developments may happen later, but when we're waiting for miracles, a year or two seems a very short time.

——————————— **1992** ———————————

**POTENT NEW ANTIREJECTION DRUG FOR TRANSPLAN-TATION APPROVED.** FK506 markedly enhances survival of transplanted organs.

**CHOLESTEROL LOWERED WITH GENE THERAPY.** Patients with hereditary deficit of LDL receptors infused with new gene. Opens door for use in others.

**PARENTS CAN NOW CHOOSE THE SEX OF THEIR CHILD BEFORE PREGNANCY.** In vitro fertilization (IVF) guarantees 100 percent accuracy.

**IMPORTANT STEP TAKEN IN DIABETES TREATMENT.** Researchers able to grow cells in laboratory that will both produce insulin and secrete it only when the body needs it. After a few improvements, will be inserted in recently developed special semi-permeable membranes. Animal tests will begin within three years.

**FIRST DRUG TO TREAT ALZHEIMER'S DISEASE AP-PROVED.** Improves symptoms by slowing down breakdown of crucial chemical messenger of which most Alzheimer's patients are deficient.

**NEW DRUG APPROVED FOR TREATING ENLARGED PROSTATES.** Merck's Proscar and other similar drugs predicted to replace most surgery within five years.

**FIRST "FEMALE CONDOM" APPROVED.** Women given a safe, cheap and easy contraceptive option.

——————————— **1993** ———————————

**ROUTINE BLOOD TESTING FOR CYSTIC FIBROSIS CAR-RIERS NOW POSSIBLE.** After the first gene was identified, it was discovered that many variations existed. Until all these variations were identified, testing for carriers was too unreliable. All genes are now identified and routine carrier testing will soon begin.

**GENETIC SCREENING DECLARED PRIVATE.** Law prohibits insurance companies, employers, from gaining access to genetic tests performed by doctors.

**ONCE-A-MONTH, SAFE, INJECTABLE CONTRACEPTIVE FOR WOMEN NOW WIDELY AVAILABLE.** Known as Cyclofem and Mesigyna, their big advantage is fewer side effects than Norplant.

**NEW SAFE TREATMENT FOR WRINKLED SKIN APPROVED.** Alpha-hydroxy acids cause fewer side effects than Retin-A.

**BREAKTHROUGH HEMOPHILIA TREATMENT AVAILABLE.** Hemophiliacs lack a clotting substance called factor VIII. Because the substitute clotting factors used to treat them are pooled from the blood of thousands of people, hemophiliacs remained at risk for HIV and other infection until monoclonal antibody purification techniques were introduced in 1990. But the latest breakthrough, the availability of genetically engineered clotting factor, completely eliminates the risk of HIV and other bloodborne viral transmission.

**BIG STEP TAKEN IN DISCOVERING INHERITANCE OF ALZHEIMER'S DISEASE.** Identification of new gene will help determine those most at risk.

**SPECIFIC TEST FOR LYME DISEASE NOW AVAILABLE.** Earlier tests only detected the presence or absence of antibodies to the bacterium that caused Lyme disease. The new test uses molecular probes to identify the genetic structure of the organism in tissue fluids. Allows for better and earlier treatment.

**STUDY TO DEFINITIVELY DETERMINE WHETHER EXCESS DIETARY FAT CAUSES BREAST CANCER BEGUN.** After many internal battles, the National Cancer Institute agrees to provide funding. Will involve thousands of women for at least five years. Should definitively resolve the fat–breast cancer connection. Part of the recent strong emphasis placed on women's health problems by National Institutes of Health director Berna-dine Healy.

**FIRST SUB-4-MINUTE MILE RUN BY FORTY-YEAR-OLD MALE.** Remarkable improvement in training techniques helps break performance barrier.

**FIFTY PERCENT OF ALL PATIENTS IMPROVED BY NEW ALZHEIMER'S DISEASE DRUGS.** Work in same way as first drugs but safer and more effective.

**INSPIRING NEWS FOR PATIENTS WITH CHRONIC FA-TIGUE SYNDROME.** Patients with chronic fatigue have immune defects, thought to be caused by a virus. Although not all of the immune problems nor the virus has been specifically identified, a drug approved in 1993, which is both antiviral and immune mod-ulating, significantly helps most patients.

**SEVERE DISEASES IN NEWBORNS GUARANTEED ELIM-INATED.** Prospective parents can use in vitro fertilization to test embryos for Tay-Sachs disease, Huntington's disease and cystic fibrosis before pregnancy.

**LUNG CANCER PROVEN TO BE GENETICALLY DETER-MINED.** Identification of first gene will help determine which smokers are at greatest risk.

# 1994

**ODDS TIPPED IN FAVOR OF COUPLES USING IN VITRO FERTILIZATION TO BECOME PREGNANT.** Culturing em-bryo in oviduct cells (cells that line the fallopian tube) before im-planting in mother's womb markedly enhances chances of success.

**RELIEF FOR ASTHMA SUFFERERS.** New drug, called a leu-kotriene antagonist, markedly improves symptoms in three of four patients. It works by getting right to the molecular source of the inflammatory process and modulating it.

**BREAKTHROUGH IN TREATING OBESITY.** Newest drug approved sustains weight loss for longest period yet. It is the latest of a class of compounds called serotonin agonists which reduce hunger. Even better drugs on target for the future.

**ANTIOXIDANT SUPPLEMENTATION SHOWN TO REDUCE RISK OF CANCER.** Most physicians begin recommending beta-carotene, vitamin C and vitamin E to their patients.

**FINALLY, A SAFE IUD APPROVED.** New device, called Flexigard, is extremely flexible and does not have the protuberances that conventional IUDs need to keep them in place within the uterine cavity. Results in far less pain or bleeding.

**A DRUG TO PREVENT BREAST CANCER.** Following large study which showed a protective effect, women at high risk urged to take tamoxifen.

**PROTEIN FRAGMENTS LINKED TO ALZHEIMER'S DISEASE.** Abnormalities in processing of amyloid may be ultimate cause.

**RISK OF HEART DISEASE AND CANCER DETERMINED BY SIMPLE BLOOD TEST.** Physicians now routinely measuring blood levels of antioxidants in their patients.

**NEW GENES FOR ALCOHOLISM PRECISELY IDENTIFIED.** Test to determine susceptibility on horizon.

**NEW HOPE FOR SCHIZOPHRENIA PATIENTS.** The drug clozapine, the most successful antischizophrenia treatment ever available, worked by blocking certain abnormal brain receptors identified in schizophrenics. The identification of additional abnormal receptor sites in the brain now opens the door for safe, new treatments.

**PATIENTS NOW ABLE TO ORDER ANY BLOOD TEST WITHOUT A DOCTOR'S PRESCRIPTION.** Direct-access laboratories declared law in all states.

**COLON CANCER DETECTED AT EARLY STAGE WITH STOOL ANALYSIS.** Test looks for mutations in important p53 gene as well as others. Predicted to save lives.

**ANOTHER CONTRACEPTIVE OPTION FOR WOMEN.** Hormone-releasing vaginal ring is long-lasting, self-installed.

**NEW AIRLINE POLICIES HELP PASSENGERS AVOID JET LAG.** European flights departing in morning; more in tune with our biological clocks.

**TRADITIONAL GALLBLADDER SURGERY PRACTICALLY OBSOLETE.** More than 80 percent of all operations now done by laparoscopy.

**NEW GUIDELINES PROMISE TO PROVIDE ADDITIONAL FUNDS FOR SCIENTIFIC RESEARCH.** Industry and universities can collaborate under strict regulation.

**"MORNING-AFTER" CONTRACEPTIVE PILL APPROVED FOR WOMEN.** Successfully tested in China, it prevents pregnancy if taken within twenty-four hours after intercourse.

**NEW CHOLESTEROL-LOWERING DRUGS THE MOST EFFECTIVE YET DEVELOPED.** Superior even to lovastatin and related drugs with fewer side effects.

**LATEST AIDS DRUG ANOTHER BREAKTHROUGH.** Prevents attachment of HIV virus to immune cells, earliest stage in infection.

—————————————— **1995** ——————————————

**BREAST "PAP SMEAR" UNVEILED, PROMISES TO SAVE MANY PATIENTS.** Called a ductogram, involves removing washings from breast ducts to look for abnormal cells at very early stage. Soon to lead to new treatment.

**NEW FOOD LABELING LAW HELPS CONSUMERS PREVENT DISEASE.** Food and Drug Administration allows manufacturers to indicate specific disease-fighting properties of foods.

**SHORTAGE OF CADAVER ORGANS FOR TRANSPLANTATION MARKEDLY ALLEVIATED.** "Presumed consent" policy allows hospital to use organs unless specifically denied before death.

**NEW BLOOD TEST IDENTIFIES PREDISPOSITION TO AL-COHOLISM.** Based on alcoholism genes, test opens door to first specific biochemical prevention and treatment.

**SCHIZOPHRENIA PATIENTS CAN NOW BE HELPED WITH MUCH SAFER AND MORE EFFECTIVE DRUGS.** Based on recent identification of new brain receptors, these drugs have fewer side effects and are cheaper than clozapine, the most commonly used drug.

**NIGHT-SHIFT WORKERS CAN NOW STAY MORE ALERT AND REDUCE RISK FOR DISEASE.** Lighting units to reset biological clocks deemed mandatory in all facilities where there are night shifts.

**BALDNESS SOON TO BE A THING OF THE PAST.** New drugs called 5-alpha-reductase inhibitors much more effective than Rogaine. Scientists promise even more treatments soon.

**CROSS-COUNTRY TRANSPORTATION OF ORGANS FOR TRANSPLANTS POSSIBLE.** Recently developed preservation solutions extend life of hearts, livers, kidneys, pancreases from hours to days. Many more lives to be saved.

**MIND-BODY THERAPIES NOW CONSIDERED MAIN-STREAM.** Physicians find patients heal better; pharmaceutical companies endorse therapies because lower dose of drugs required leads to fewer side effects and greater compliance.

**SEVERAL FITNESS CLUBS NOW RESTRICT MEMBERSHIP TO THOSE OVER FIFTY YEARS OLD.** All equipment (weights, shoes) designed for the older exerciser.

**CORONARY BYPASS OPERATIONS DECREASED BY 50 PERCENT.** Less invasive procedures becoming the standard. Predicted to decrease even further.

**AT LAST! AN EFFECTIVE BIRTH CONTROL OPTION FOR THOSE OPPOSED TO CONTRACEPTION.** Jet-age rhythm method uses home urine test to precisely determine time of ovulation.

**ARTHRITIS SLOWED BY NEW DRUG.** Inhibits cysteine, a faulty amino acid (building block of joint tissue) in patients with osteoarthritis gene.

**IMPORTANT STEP IN CANCER TREATMENT.** Laboratory synthesis of Taxol, the very effective drug previously available only from the bark of the yew tree, means abundant supply and help for thousands with ovarian and other cancers.

**CANCER THERAPY TAILORED TO INDIVIDUAL PATIENTS.** Blood test measures presence or absence of oncogenes (cancer-activating genes) or antioncogenes (cancer-suppressing genes), helps determine dosage of chemotherapy.

**HIGH-TECH FOODS HELP PREVENT DISEASE.** Supermarkets begin carrying "nutriceuticals," foods biotechnologically enhanced with specific disease-fighting properties.

**DOCTORS NOW PERFORM FETAL SURGERY ROUTINELY.** Once an experimental procedure, operating on unborn still in the womb saves many babies.

## —— 1996 ——

**ALL MAJOR U.S. CORPORATIONS NOW USE ENVIRONMENTALLY SAFE MANUFACTURING PROCESSES.** New chemical processes keep up production without harming our health.

**IMPORTANT FIRST STEP TAKEN TOWARD UNIVERSAL HEALTH INSURANCE.** "Smart cards" issued to everyone, to be used in all physician and hospital visits. Will result in huge national data bank of risks and benefits of every medical procedure.

**"NO-SCALPEL" VASECTOMY AVAILABLE FOR MEN.** Two new options, successfully tested in China and the Third World, will replace traditional vasectomies. In one, a tiny puncture hole is made in the skin, the sperm ducts clamped with a special forceps and then exposed and tied off. In the other, a solution is injected directly into the sperm ducts and then hardens and blocks passage of sperm. Both methods are easy to perform and reverse.

**BABIES BORN WITHOUT BRAINS APPROVED AS ORGAN DONORS.** Since these children, called anencephalic infants, always die within a few weeks, it allows for some good to come from a tragic situation.

**AIRLINES TAKE ANOTHER STEP TO HELP PASSENGERS COMBAT JET LAG.** Special lighting units installed in planes help reset travelers' biological clocks in flight.

**NOVEL PAIN MEDICATION COMES FROM RESEARCH ON MARIJUANA.** Receptors in brain for THC—the active ingredient in marijuana—identified in 1990 provide key to drug development.

**EXCITING NEW DRUGS APPROVED FOR TREATMENT OF HYPERTENSION.** Manipulation of vascular growth factors hailed as a breakthrough.

**HOPE FOR LUNG CANCER PATIENTS.** Molecular diagnostic test on sputum picks up mutations in p53 gene, catching tumor at early, curable stage.

**INNOVATION IN BREAST CANCER SURGERY A BOON TO PATIENTS.** Research reveals that removing only affected ducts rather than larger part of the breast is even more effective treatment, and not disfiguring at all.

**ANIMAL TESTING OF DRUGS AND COSMETICS COMPLETELY ELIMINATED.** Replaced by much more humane computer modeling and cell cultures.

**PATIENT ACTIVISTS HAVE MAJOR IMPACT IN APPROVAL OF CANCER AND ALZHEIMER'S DISEASE TREATMENTS.** Taking lead from AIDS activists, newly organized groups strongly influence FDA processes and help new treatments become available earlier.

**FIRST NEW ALLERGY TREATMENT IN YEARS OFFERS REAL HOPE FOR SUFFERERS.** Drugs and monoclonal antibodies block attachment of the allergy-producing substances to the susceptible cells in the body.

# 1997

**BUYING AND SELLING OF LIVE ORGANS LEGALIZED.** Unprecedented move designed to alleviate organ shortage for transplant and circumvent unscrupulous "organ brokers." Will be closely regulated and tax deductible.

**NEW ALZHEIMER'S DRUG BEGINS TO ADDRESS CAUSE.** Increases chemical called substance P which antagonizes protein fragment toxic to the brain.

**A GENUINE CURE FOR CRIPPLING MUSCULAR DYSTROPHY.** Genetic therapy introduces normal genes to muscle cells.

**A NEW CHEMOPREVENTIVE FOR BREAST CANCER.** 4-HPR, a synthetic vitamin A derivative, proves safe and effective in clinical trials. Added to effects of tamoxifen, risk of breast cancer is decreased even further.

**VACCINE FOR LYME DISEASE APPROVED.** Highly effective, recommended for everyone.

**COLON CANCER ON THE WAY OUT.** Genetic mechanisms fully elucidated. Earlier detection than ever and complete prevention to come within ten to fifteen years.

**IMPOTENCE ELIMINATED FOR GOOD.** Injection of vascular factors (endothelins) provide successful treatment.

**ANOTHER POWERFUL ANTIREJECTION DRUG APPROVED FOR TRANSPLANT PATIENTS.** Rapamycin works together with FK506 to prolong organ survival even further.

**HEART DISEASE PREVENTED BY VITAMINS.** Vitamin E, beta-carotene and powerful new antioxidants routinely prescribed by doctors.

**ABORTION DRUG APPROVED IN UNITED STATES.** Evidence on RU-486 from other countries could no longer be ignored. A victory for pro-choice.

**ALZHEIMER'S DISEASE CAN FINALLY BE DIAGNOSED ACCURATELY.** Blood test for a specific protein and two noninvasive imaging tests (PET and SPECT) provide the answers.

**LONG-STANDING SPEED BARRIER BROKEN.** First sub-3:40 mile incredible human performance achievement.

**FIRST AIDS VACCINE APPROVED.** Hailed as a breakthrough in AIDS prevention. Even more to come in prevention and treatment.

**EIGHT OF TEN ALZHEIMER'S PATIENTS IMPROVED WITH LATEST DRUGS.** Newest generation of compounds most effective yet. Address combination of neurotransmitter defects.

**THE END OF DENTURES.** New titanium implants and better computer design allow for permanent replacement of teeth.

**PARKINSON'S DISEASE CONTROLLABLE WITH GENETIC ENGINEERING.** Laboratory-grown brain cells manipulated to produce dopamine, the chemical Parkinson's patients lack, and then transplanted into the brain.

**DEPRESSION NOW COMPLETELY MANAGEABLE BIO-CHEMICALLY.** Discovery of more receptor sites in brain leads to development of drugs more sophisticated, more effective and safer than Prozac.

**ALL WOMEN CAN NOW BE TESTED FOR OSTEOPOROSIS IN THEIR DOCTOR'S OFFICE.** Test is simple and cheap, no more difficult than having blood pressure taken.

**NO MORE AGE BARRIERS ON HIP AND KNEE REPLACE-MENT.** Ten-year life-span of replacements previously limited them to older people, but latest extended-wear synthetic biomaterials last more than twice as long.

**UNLIKELY SOURCE ALLOWS PATIENTS TO MONITOR HEALTH AT HOME.** High-tech toilet performs urinalysis, measures blood pressure, weight and fat percentage. Available in most homes.

**MOST EYEGLASSES NO LONGER NECESSARY.** Laser sculpting of cornea eliminates 75 percent of nearsightedness.

**LONG-PROMISED CANCER VACCINE APPROVED.** Important breakthrough for kidney cancer and malignant melanoma, but different strategies being developed for other cancers.

**DOCTORS CAN NOW WATCH OVER THEIR PATIENTS FROM AFAR.** Ordinary-looking plastic watches continually monitor heart rate, blood pressure and brain waves and call doctor if there is an abnormality.

**CANCER PATIENTS TREATED MORE EFFECTIVELY AND SAFELY WITH IMPLANTABLE DRUG DELIVERY SYSTEMS.** Biosensors and computers monitor cancer cell division as determined by biological clock. Kills more cancer cells, with far fewer side effects.

**SUPERMARKET SHOPPING CARTS LIAISON BETWEEN PATIENTS AND DOCTORS.** Equipped with interactive computers, patients can punch in lab results and get menus tailored to their health profile.

**EFFECTS OF AGING REVERSED BY INJECTION.** Recombinant growth hormone approved after years of research. Promises more muscle, better skin for elderly.

—————————— **1998** ——————————

**WOMEN HAVING BABIES AT ANY AGE NOW POSSIBLE.** New developments in freezing and thawing of embryos allows women to have an egg fertilized when younger, to have the embryo stored frozen and to become pregnant whenever they want.

**IMPORTANT BREAKTHROUGH FOR COUPLES USING IN VITRO FERTILIZATION.** A protein "glue" that aids implantation of embryo in the uterus now available as a drug; predicted to dramatically increase success of procedure.

**DRUG OVERDOSES REVERSED BY MOLECULAR BIOLOGY IN EMERGENCY ROOM.** Injection of catalytic antibodies, a combination of antibodies and enzymes, bind to drug and change it to nontoxic form.

**BIRTH CONTROL VACCINE PREVENTS PREGNANCY FOR AN ENTIRE YEAR.** The ultimate contraceptive, only one injection of anti-hCG (human chorionic gonadotropin) required.

**ANXIETY CAN NOW BE TREATED WITHOUT DEPENDENCY.** New drugs even more effective than Valium and with no addictive potential.

**ALL AMERICANS FINALLY GUARANTEED UNIVERSAL HEALTH INSURANCE.** New plan unique, paid for by combination of government, employer's and patient's own funds, depending on one's situation.

**PARENTS OF NEWBORNS GIVEN PEACE OF MIND WITH "SIDS MATTRESS."** Sudden infant death syndrome prevented by sensors impregnated into the crib mattress which continually monitor infant's vital signs and sound alarm if anything goes wrong.

**JET-LAG TREATMENT BECOMES PORTABLE.** Lighting units for resetting biological clocks now compact and lightweight. Used by international travelers, mobile night-shift workers (policemen, truckers).

**BALDNESS NOW TREATED BY MOLECULAR BIOLOGY.** New drugs and monoclonal antibodies remarkably effective, block attachment to cell receptors of baldness-inducing hormone dihydroxytestosterone.

**NEW HOPE FOR PATIENTS WITH LOW LEVELS OF HDL CHOLESTEROL.** First drugs to directly raise HDL cholesterol predicted to prevent thousands of heart attacks each year.

**TESTING FINDS IT DANGEROUS TO SOCIETY, THEMSELVES, FOR SOME PEOPLE TO WORK AT NIGHT.** Lack of adaptability of their biological clocks to light treatments brands them "chronobiologically unemployable."

**FIRST SUB-2-HOUR MARATHON RUN BY MALE.** Barrier thought to be impossible shattered by high-tech training methods and equipment.

**RISK OF SKIN CANCER IN SUN WORSHIPPERS MARKEDLY REDUCED.** DNA repair enzymes derived from viruses can repair sun-damaged skin.

**BREAST CANCER TREATED WITH LASERS.** Abnormal cells detected on breast "Pap" removed before tumor can grow.

**GALLBLADDER SURGERY FOR GALLSTONES OUTMODED.** Even most laparoscopic surgery replaced by drugs and shock waves. Complete prevention of gallstones forecast for 2000.

**NEW VACCINE ELIMINATES CAVITIES.** Immunizes against bacteria that cause dental caries. Fluoride no longer needed.

**STROKE VICTIMS CAN LOOK FORWARD TO FAR BETTER RESULT.** Drugs called lazaroids and glutamate receptor blockers given shortly after stroke prevent permanent damage.

**CORONARY ARTERY DISEASE NOW DIAGNOSED WITHOUT GOING INTO THE HOSPITAL.** New noninvasive angiogram completely safe and done on outpatient basis.

**ALZHEIMER'S PATIENTS HELPED BY GENETIC ENGINEERING.** Scientists transplant laboratory-grown brain cells spliced with gene for acetylcholine, an important chemical deficient in the brains of Alzheimer's patients. Seventy-five percent of patients treated improved.

**CATARACTS PREVENTED BY ANTIOXIDANTS.** Leading cause of blindness worldwide declines 75 percent with international distribution of vitamins C, E, beta-carotene.

# 1999

**BALDNESS REVERSED BY TRANSPLANTING HAIR FOLLICLES GROWN IN THE LABORATORY.** No more painful and unnatural hair "plugs." Abundant supply for those who didn't get baldness-treatment drugs soon enough.

**LUNG CANCER RISK CLEARLY DEFINABLE.** Scientists declare that all predisposing genes are identifiable. Opens door for simple test within two years.

**SPREAD OF CANCER CAN NOW BE TIGHTLY CONTROLLED.** New drug that inhibits metastasis gene approved. Predicted to lead to significant increase in survival.

**ANOTHER MAJOR BREAKTHOUGH IN IN VITRO FERTILIZATION.** New technological development biochemically analyzes embryo before implantation to predict viability.

**ARTIFICIAL SKIN A GODSEND FOR BURN VICTIMS.** Grown in laboratory, solves shortage of suitable skin for grafting. Predicted to be used for cosmetic purposes within three years.

**CLEANING OUT ARTERIES AS AN OUTPATIENT.** New techniques—laser angioplasty and atherectomy—markedly improved and simplified. Patients go home the same day.

**SURGERY NO LONGER TREATMENT OF CHOICE FOR PROSTATE CANCER.** New drugs just as effective without the side effects of surgery.

## 2000

**TRANSPLANTS NOW POSSIBLE WITHOUT ANTIREJECTION DRUGS.** Pretransplant procedure called immunological tolerance leads to perfect donor-recipient matches and no risk of infection.

**SIMPLE BLOOD TEST IDENTIFIES THOSE WITH LUNG CANCER PREDISPOSITION.** Pinpoints all genes that render one susceptible. Opens door for manipulation within ten years.

**FINALLY WINNING THE WAR ON CANCER.** Treatments introduced in past ten years have decreased overall incidence 35 percent and death 50 percent. Advances in specific cancers even greater. Much more progress predicted for future.

**MORE PROGRESS AGAINST AIDS.** New drugs called protease inhibitors and antisense oligonucleotides, along with already proven methods, stop HIV in several sites. Incidence in developed countries down 50 percent.

**SUCCESSFUL ATTACK ON PERIODONTAL DISEASE.** Inflammation stopped with drugs called prostaglandin modulators, bone restored with growth factors.

**MASTERS' POWER.** First sub-4-minute mile run by fifty-year-old male.

**PATIENTS HELPED BY NEW APPROACH TO DRUG DEVELOPMENT.** All new drugs now designed by computer and produced by biotechnology. Faster and more specific.

**CORONARY BYPASS SURGERY DECREASED BY 75 PERCENT.** Most patients now have outpatient procedures. Still used for multiple bypass.

**FIRST DRUG TO PREVENT GALLSTONES.** Called antinucleating drugs, stop accumulation of cholesterol, other substances in gallbladder. Forecast to eliminate most gallstones.

**MOST U.S. PHYSICIANS NO LONGER WHITE MALES.** Women, minorities now compose more than 50 percent.

**BONES WEAKENED BY OSTEOPOROSIS REBUILT.** Substance developed by biotechnology mimics parathyroid hormone, safely increases bone mass and strength.

**CURE RATE OF PROSTATE CANCER INCREASED BY 50 PERCENT.** Blood test responsible for early detection in more men.

**MEMORY IMPROVED WITH DRUGS.** Only used for Alzheimer's patients now, but other exciting applications soon.

**THE DEATH OF THE PRIVATE PRACTITIONER.** Two of three physicians now practice in HMOs.

**REVOLUTIONARY REVISION OF RDA FOR VITAMINS.** New research on protective effects of antioxidant vitamins against cancer, heart disease convinces Food and Drug Administration to increase RDAs for vitamin E, C.

## 2001

**A GIANT PERFORMANCE STEP FOR WOMEN.** First sub-2:15 marathon run by a female.

**HOME BIRTHS PERFORMED BY PARENTS.** High-tech monitoring from physician's office allows parents to safely deliver their own children.

**MOST EFFECTIVE TREATMENT YET FOR RHEUMATOID ARTHRITIS.** Biotechnology develops treatment to block inflammation. The new drugs work at several stages of the inflammatory process, at the level of the immune cells, the blood capillaries and the vulnerable joints. Represents the strongest promise yet to dramatically relieve symptoms.

**AGING SLOWED BY NEW VITAMINS.** Called PQQ and BH4, interfere with cell's genetic clock; will be available for purchase within ten years.

**AN INCREDIBLE BREAKTHROUGH FOR CYSTIC FIBROSIS PATIENTS.** This previously untreatable and fatal disease is now controllable with genetic therapy. The lifesaving genes that cystic fibrosis patients are missing are now delivered by means of an aerosol inhaled at approximately monthly intervals. Will allow them to live completely normal lives.

**BIRTH CONTROL PILL FOR MALES FINALLY ARRIVES.** Regulates level of testosterone, and therefore sperm production, without affecting libido.

**A SHOCKING NEW SOURCE OF ORGANS FOR TRANSPLANTATION.** Some parents use advanced reproductive technology to "create" anencephalic infants. Future breakthroughs will make this only a temporary solution.

# 2002

**NO MORE WRINKLES.** Artificial skin, previously used for burn patients, improved and now indistinguishable from natural. Used for cosmetic purposes.

**ALCOHOLISM BIOCHEMICALLY TREATABLE AT LAST.** Designer substances called "brain vitamins" correct abnormal genes, individualize treatment.

**CORONARY ARTERY DISEASE DOWN 50 PERCENT; DEATH RATE DOWN 70 PERCENT.** Outpatient diagnostic and treatment techniques, along with better prevention, cited as reasons. Even more progress to come.

**AIDS EPIDEMIC HALTED.** Genetic therapy and "genetic antibiotics" decrease incidence, increase cure 80 percent.

**OSTEOPOROSIS PREVENTED BY DRUG THAT REPLACES ESTROGEN.** Designed by computer to be as effective as estrogen but without increasing risk of breast cancer.

**CANCER TREATMENT MAINSTAYS NO LONGER SURGERY, RADIATION AND CHEMOTHERAPY.** Biotherapy, which works with patient's own defenses, more individualized, safer and effective. Surpasses other treatments in use.

**EUTHANASIA LEGALIZED.** Political pressure from aging baby-boomers forces decision.

**LUNG CANCER INCIDENCE REDUCED 35 PERCENT; DEATH RATE DECREASED 45 PERCENT.** Result of molecular diagnostics and antismoking programs, but bigger breakthroughs to come soon.

# 2003

**TRANSPLANTATION GAINS FROM AN UNLIKELY SOURCE.** Use of animal organs, called xenografts, made possible by the new antirejection drugs that allows for interspecies organ sharing.

**ALLERGY TREATMENT IMPROVED.** By biotechnologically modifying the immune response, treatment made more specific and effective.

**ALL DIABETES GENES IDENTIFIED.** Opens door for molecular prevention at early age.

**COURSE OF ALZHEIMER'S DISEASE ACTUALLY SLOWED.** More than just treating symptoms, new generation of drugs stops damage and stimulates growth of cells; 85 percent of patients improve.

**STOMACH AND PANCREATIC CANCERS NO LONGER DEADLY.** Early detection with ultrasound and SPECT imaging, treatment with lasers make them manageable.

# 2004

**MOTHER-CHILD BONDING HORMONE CLARIFIED.** Identification of specific part of oxytocin molecule opens door for amazing parental options.

**HEREDITY OF HEART DISEASE DETERMINED.** All predisposing genes identified. Will lead to testing within two years and preventive therapy within ten years.

**PREDISPOSITION TO ALL ADDICTIONS DETERMINED.** Abnormal "pleasure-seeking" genes identified in cocaine, heroin, nicotine addiction, obesity. Specific diagnostic techniques and treatments soon available.

**THE TWENTY-FIRST CENTURY HOUSE CALL.** Using fiberoptic technology, patients can have video appointments with their doctors without leaving home.

**MEMORY BOOST FOR OLDER PEOPLE.** Drugs used previously to improve memory in Alzheimer's patients approved for normal age-related memory loss.

**REVERSING THE ENGINE OF CANCER.** A major breakthrough in cancer treatment: tumor suppressor genes added to leukemia cells, convert them to normal blood cells. To be used for solid tumors within nine years.

**HEART TRANSPLANTS REPLACED BY SOMETHING BETTER.** Totally implantable artificial heart works perfectly, available over-the-counter.

**TREATING JET LAG AND SLEEP DISORDERS WITH A NEW PILL.** Supplements of the hormone melatonin readjust biological clock. Easier to use than light.

**BIG STEP TOWARD ALZHEIMER'S PREVENTION.** Scientists identify final gene. Testing and prevention to begin within four years.

# 2005

**FIRST GROUP OF ALZHEIMER'S PATIENTS CURED.** New growth factors and combination drugs actually cure 35 percent of patients. Just the beginning.

**HOPE FOR MORE CANCER PATIENTS.** Genes that predispose to prostate and breast cancer identified. Tests to identify and then therapies to manipulate genes available soon.

**STROKE DAMAGE REVERSAL POSSIBLE.** Nerve growth factors aid in repairing brain cells. Residual effects to be kept to minimum.

**ARTIFICIAL PANCREAS PERFECTED.** Insulin-producing and -secreting cells successfully tested in animals and humans. Ready for routine clinical use. Expected to markedly reduce diabetic complications.

**ALLERGIES EFFECTIVELY ELIMINATED.** Complete understanding of cellular cascade-causing allergic symptoms leads to molecular compounds to nip it in the bud.

**SCHIZOPHRENIA PATIENTS TO BENEFIT FROM MOLECULAR BIOLOGY.** Newest drugs target brain receptor deficits more effectively. Fifty percent improvement expected.

**INCREDIBLE: BLOOD TESTS WITHOUT DRAWING BLOOD.** Patients perform themselves and send results to doctors. Ear clips with lasers map structure of compounds in capillaries.

**BALDNESS TREATED WITH GENETIC THERAPY.** The ultimate treatment, manipulates gene that regulates baldness enzyme.

**SURGERY FOR BREAST CANCER OBSOLETE.** Breast Pap smears and lasers eliminate early problems; later problems treated with biological response modifiers.

**CARDIOVASCULAR DISEASE TREATED WITH ANOTHER GENETIC THERAPY ADVANCE.** Manipulating endothelial cells (that line blood vessels) prevents blockages from occurring.

**AGING SLOWED BY NEW DRUG.** Inhibits age-related uncoiling of DNA in cell. Predicted to increase life-span.

**JOINT SURGERY FOR ARTHRITIS DISCARDED FOR MOLECULAR THERAPY.** Cartilage growth enhancers more effective and permanent than hip and knee replacement.

## 2006

**RHEUMATOID ARTHRITIS TREATED BY IMMUNIZATION.** Vaccination against traitorous T-cells prevents progress of disease.

**HEART DISEASE PREDISPOSITION IDENTIFIED BY BLOOD TEST.** Detects all genes that determine susceptibility. Allows for early prevention.

**GENETICS OF RHEUMATOID ARTHRITIS UNRAVELED.** Complex set of genes fully identified. Opens door for diagnostic blood test and eventual prevention.

**SURROGATE PARENTING NOW A DEFINABLE CAREER FOR MANY WOMEN.** Live in "surrogate spas" while pregnant; diet, lifestyle carefully controlled.

**ADDICTION GENES NOW DETECTABLE.** Simple blood test identifies all abnormal "pleasure-seeking" genes. Prevention and treatment possible next year.

# 2007

**THE NEXT PLAGUE: EPIDEMIOLOGISTS DECLARE NEW VIRAL EPIDEMIC.** Caused by activation of a normally harmless virus. The result of man's manipulation of his environment.

**DRUG ADDICTION CONQUERED, SMOKELESS SOCIETY FINALLY ACHIEVED.** Designer drugs correct abnormal genes, eliminate desire.

**SLEEPING ONLY NINETY MINUTES A DAY PREVENTS ACCIDENTS, SAVES LIVES.** Polyphasic sleep works with biological clock. Helps medical residents, fire fighters, space station workers. Not to be used by everyone.

**PERIODONTAL DISEASE PREVENTABLE.** New polyvalent vaccine (against several bacteria) provides protection.

**NEGATIVE SYMPTOMS OF SCHIZOPHRENIA NOW TREATABLE.** Eliminate residual antisocial feelings after hallucinations treated. Major advance allows patients to return to meaningful life. Much more to come.

**EXTENDING THE LIMITS OF HUMAN LIFESPAN.** Multiple mechanisms of aging well-understood, including genetic ones. Intervention will lead to human living well beyond one hundred twenty years.

## 2008

**PARENTAL BONDING NOW BIOCHEMICALLY CONTROL-LABLE.** Drugs mimicking or blocking actions of bonding hormone oxytocin eliminates problems with surrogate mothers.

**GUARANTEED PERFECTLY HEALTHY BABIES NOW A VI-ABLE OPTION.** Possible to test embryos created by in vitro fertilization for predisposition to cancer, heart disease, several others.

**BUYING BODY PARTS OFF THE SHELF.** Totally implantable artificial kidneys, livers, pancreases, purchased over-the-counter and coated with recipient's genetic code.

**ACCURATELY PREDICTING WHO MIGHT DEVELOP ALZ-HEIMER'S DISEASE.** Blood test detects presence of all abnormal predisposing genes. Preventive manipulation of genes soon available.

**MAJOR ADVANCE IN PREVENTION OF SCHIZOPHRE-NIA.** All genes identified. Testing soon.

**ULCERATIVE COLITIS AND CROHN'S DISEASE SUCCESS-FULLY TREATED WITH GENE THERAPY.** Through the use of drugs that correct the molecular defect in intestinal cells, this therapy at last provides a genuine cure for both of these devastating diseases previously treated only at the symptomatic level.

## 2009

**AT LAST! COLDS CAN BE PREVENTED.** Polyvalent vaccine (against most common cold–causing viruses) prevents 80 percent of colds. Better antiviral drugs available for treatment, but short duration of colds makes use impractical.

**FIRST ARTIFICIAL BRAIN INTRODUCED.** Doesn't duplicate all functions of brain, just memory. More elaborate brains predicted.

**SCIENCE FACT, NOT FICTION. FIRST HUMAN SUCCESSFULLY CLONED!** Purpose is for repository of organs for transplantation, but possible to use to indefinitely extend life.

**HEALING FRACTURES IN A WEEK.** All kinks worked out of electromagnetic induction. Works for regenerating nerves as well as bone.

**ALL NEWBORN BABIES TESTED FOR DISEASE SUSCEPTIBILITIES.** Genetic testing results to remain private. Used for early prevention.

**GENES THAT DETERMINE ABILITIES AND TALENTS IDENTIFIED.** Leaves door open for designer babies.

## 2010

**GENETIC SUSCEPTIBILITIES FOR CANCER REVERSED.** Drugs designed by molecular biology manipulate faulty genes for lung and colon cancer. The ultimate in prevention.

**A MIRACLE FOR PARAPLEGICS AND QUADRIPLEGICS.** Artificial nerves bypass spinal cord breaks. Complete recovery for crippled patients.

**SPENDING OLD AGE IN HAPPINESS.** Breakthroughs in brain chemistry allow elderly to have pleasurable experiences without side effects.

**OSTEOPOROSIS TREATMENT ADVANCES FURTHER.** Cytokines, other growth factors superior to bone-building drugs. Problem eliminated within ten years.

**CREATING "SUPERNORMAL" MEMORIES.** Drugs used previously for Alzheimer's, normal elderly, now used on teenagers and adults. Controversial enhancement therapy.

**VARIETY OF NEW POSSIBILITIES FOR CREATING BABIES.** Successful freezing of human eggs allows for many different in vitro fertilization options, not just for infertile couples.

**ALZHEIMER'S DISEASE TREATMENT TAKES ANOTHER STEP TOWARD CURE.** Designer drugs interfere with molecular cascade that causes abnormal amyloid protein. Ninety percent improve, half cured. One more major breakthrough to come.

**SCHIZOPHRENIA CLOSE TO BEING PREVENTABLE.** Simple blood test able to identify all predisposing genes. Manipulation soon possible.

**BIOLOGICAL CLOCKS RESET WITH NEW DRUGS.** Neurotransmitter compounds can manipulate effectively in any direction. No more "chronobiologically unemployable."

**INCIDENCE OF CORONARY ARTERY DISEASE DECREASED 75 PERCENT; DEATH RATE DECREASED BY 85 PERCENT.** Molecular diagnostics responsible for early prevention. Latest breakthrough in manipulation of genetic susceptibilities will eliminate almost completely within twenty years.

**CANCER NO LONGER MAJOR THREAT.** Incidence down 65 percent; death rate down 75 percent. Further application of molecular biology will provide even greater decline.

## 2011

**PICKING UP CANCER AT EARLIEST POSSIBLE LEVEL.** New test can diagnose one gene mutation in ten billion cells. Easily reversible before any damage occurs.

**PRAYING FOR PATIENTS.** Application of quantum physics principle of nonlocality improves recovery. Physicians risk malpractice suit if they don't enlist prayer groups for patients.

**AVERAGE LIFE EXPECTANCY AT BIRTH REACHES NINETY YEARS.** Breakthroughs in cancer, cardiovascular disease, aging responsible. Will increase more.

**CORONARY BYPASS SURGERY DECREASED BY 95 PER-CENT.** Molecular biology and genetic therapy prevent most cases; others treated as outpatients.

**AUTOIMMUNE DISEASE COMPLETELY CONTROLLABLE.** Predisposing genes identified at birth, and abnormal immune cells eliminated by monoclonal antibodies. Prevents rheumatoid arthritis, multiple sclerosis, myasthenia gravis, systemic lupus.

## 2012

**INCIDENCE OF PROSTATE CANCER DECREASED 70 PER-CENT, DEATH RATE BY 80 PERCENT.** Early detection, molecular therapy responsible.

**ARTIFICIAL LIMBS REACH PERFECTION.** Look and function like natural arms and legs. Combine with artificial nerves to restore normality to trauma victims.

**COMPLETE PREVENTION OF SCHIZOPHRENIA CLOSE.** All risk factors causing gene expression identified. With genetic therapy, possible to totally prevent within five years.

**GENETIC TESTING FOR ABILITIES AVAILABLE.** Opens door for biochemically creating smart, talented babies, changing abilities after birth.

**BREAKTHROUGH IN ARTIFICIAL ORGANS.** Eyes and ears, look real, function even better than natural sensory organs.

## 2013

**INCIDENCE OF COLON CANCER DECREASED 75 PER-CENT; DEATH RATE DECREASED 90 PERCENT.**

**BIONIC ATHLETES.** Artificial knees, ligaments and muscles for professional athletes introduced. With capabilities superior to natural versions, promise to change sports.

**TURNING CANCER CELLS INTO NORMAL ONES.** Tumor suppressor genes delivered directly to tumor by molecules called fusion proteins reverse course of cancer.

## — 2014 —

**INCIDENCE OF BREAST CANCER DECREASED 75 PERCENT; DEATH RATE DECREASED 90 PERCENT.**

**LUNG CANCER INCIDENCE REDUCED 75 PERCENT; DEATH RATE DECREASED 85 PERCENT.**

**PARENTS CAN NOW CREATE DESIGNER CHILDREN BEFORE, AFTER BIRTH.** Genetic therapy now available to manipulate genes for abilities, intelligence in preembryos as part of in vitro fertilization, or gene-altering drugs can be given after birth.

## — 2015 —

**COMPLETE BIOCHEMICAL CONTROL OVER MENTAL PROCESSES NOW POSSIBLE.** Safe substances to enhance creativity, instill confidence, selectively enhance or blunt all emotions introduced.

**THE ULTIMATE TREATMENT FOR ALZHEIMER'S DISEASE: PREVENTION.** Drugs available to prevent expression of predisposing genes. Combined with already available treatments, promise to wipe out condition.

**CORONARY HEART DISEASE BECOMES A RARE CONDITION.** Molecular approach responsible for 85 percent decrease in incidence, 95 percent decrease in death.

**THE ULTIMATE SEPARATION OF SEX AND REPRODUCTION.** Introduction of artificial placenta, combined with in vitro fertilization, allows for reproduction from conception to birth completely outside human body.

# 2020

**INCIDENCE OF ALZHEIMER'S DISEASE DECREASED BY 95 PERCENT.**

**TWENTY-FIRST CENTURY HOSPITAL SHARP CONTRAST FROM PREVIOUS ONES.** With chronic disease well under control, no longer need for large institutions. Now much smaller, mostly automated. Robots, laser manipulators perform many operations.

**MOST CONDITIONS CAN NOW BE DIAGNOSED AND TREATED AT HOME.** New generation of noninvasive imaging equipment simple to use at home. Diseases detected at cell level, eliminated by orally administered, genetically engineered compounds.

**INCIDENCE OF ALL CANCER DECREASED BY 80 PERCENT; DEATH RATE DECREASED BY 90 PERCENT.**

**INCIDENCE OF PROSTATE CANCER DECREASED 90 PERCENT; DEATH RATE FROM PROSTATE CANCER DECREASED 95 PERCENT.**

**INCIDENCE OF COLON CANCER DECREASED 90 PERCENT; DEATH RATE DECREASED 95 PERCENT.**

# 2025

**LUNG CANCER INCIDENCE REDUCED 80 PERCENT; DEATH RATE DECREASED 90 PERCENT.**

**ACHIEVING IMMORTALITY?** Cloning technology refined and cheap enough to be used routinely for extra body parts for everyone. Replace worn-out one with new version.

**AVERAGE LIFE EXPECTANCY AT BIRTH 100 YEARS.**

# —— **2030** ——

**CORONARY DISEASE, CANCER EFFECTIVELY WIPED OUT.** Cases so rare now newsworthy. Incidence, death rate down 99 percent.

**MAXIMUM HUMAN LIFE-SPAN INCREASED TO 150 YEARS.** Scientists predict more manipulation of genetic clocks to increase life-span to greater than 200 years by 2050.

# PART III

# MAJOR ILLNESSES AND MINOR CONDITIONS

# 6

# The Conquest of Cancer

NOWHERE ARE THE FRUITS OF MOLECULAR THERAPY GOING TO be more evident than in the prevention, diagnosis and treatment of cancer. Presently, one million new cases of cancer are diagnosed each year and almost five hundred thousand people die of it. By 2000, the incidence of cancer of all types will decline by 30 percent and more than two thirds of all patients will be cured. Ten years later, by 2010, cancer incidence will have declined by 60 percent and more than four of every five cases will be cured. And by 2020, more than 90 percent of cancer will be prevented and cured. Not only will cancer no longer be a feared condition, but it will be a rare one as well.

Although cancer has been with us for thousands of years, the future of cancer management began only fifteen years ago. The number of scientific advances in the understanding of normal cell metabolism (and how it goes awry in cancer) that have been made in such a brief time is staggering. And it is because of them that we can now foresee with complete confidence the demise of cancer as a threat to society. Detecting these changes at the molecular level and intervening in the process at the appropriate time are going to be the mainstay of cancer prevention, diagnosis and treatment by 1999. Until we reach that point, progress in our fight against cancer will depend on further achievements in advanced imaging techniques, immunological diagnosis and treatment, and hormonal therapy.

## ───────── THE DECLINE OF BREAST CANCER ─────────

A few months ago, I drove to the airport to pick up our dear friend Claudia, visiting us from Lausanne, Switzerland. She had just received a promotion to vice-president of a major energy company in Switzerland and had arranged to take a week off to celebrate achieving a career goal she had been working toward for five years. We hadn't seen her in two years and I looked forward to a wonderful week.

She looked tired to me when I greeted her and seemed uncharacteristically quiet while we waited for her baggage. I assumed it was just jet lag. But as soon as we were in the car driving toward our home, I knew something more than that was wrong. Claudia's beautiful smile, her intelligence and her manner of speaking were so uplifting she never failed to make me feel good. But not today.

"Claudia, is there something wrong?" I asked, after two or three minutes of silence.

"I can't wait to see Liz," Claudia said, "but I'm glad you came to get me alone. It's not that I want to keep anything from her, but I have a medical problem that's scaring me so, I haven't had a good night's sleep in two weeks. And I'd rather talk to just you about it, at least for now. I thought getting that promotion was the most important thing in the world to me, but now I wonder if I'm going to live long enough to enjoy it."

Claudia was thirty-eight years old, and as far as I knew had been in perfect health, so this came completely out of left field to me. "What the hell are you talking about?" I said. "You never told me there was anything wrong with you."

"You know how close-mouthed and stoic we Swiss can be, Jeff, especially to those we care about. I just didn't want to burden you with my problems."

"Well, burden me now."

"I guess I should have asked your advice earlier. Last month, I had a lumpectomy on my left breast. It was a cancer. And now I have to take radiation treatments."

I was caught completely off guard. I was furious with Claudia for having kept this from us, her best friends, especially when one of them was a physician. But she was now so visibly shaken, this obviously wasn't the time to deal with it.

"What a horrible ordeal for you," I said. "But I'm sure your doctors told you that if the tumor was small enough to be handled by a lumpectomy and radiation, your chances of being completely cured are close to ninety percent. That's the truth, you know."

"I know," she said. "But something else I never told you is my poor mother's history. Twenty years ago, when she was only forty, she had a mastectomy. Six years ago, she had to have a hysterectomy for cancer of the cervix. And just three months ago, she started coughing up blood and her doctor discovered inoperable lung cancer. She wasn't even a smoker. How could this have happened? The doctors tell me that because of my mother's history, even though they caught my breast cancer early, there's a good chance it will recur."

"Look," I said, "What you've been told in a sense is right. Because of your family history, there's statistically more of a chance that you could get cancer again in the same breast, or in the other breast. But that's by no means the only possibility. And the way research in breast cancer, and cancer in general, is going, each year, maybe even each month, the chances of picking up a tumor early and curing it completely or detecting it even before it becomes a tumor get better and better. Claudia, I'm willing to bet you're going to live to be a happy old lady."

I explained to Claudia that, because of her family history, she could have inherited some damage to a tumor suppressor gene known as p53. p53 genes are present in all our cells, and when they work right, they act as a brake against uncontrolled cell growth. A damaged p53 is called a mutation. When a mutation loses its ability to stop the cell from growing too fast, the end result can be cancer. Factors other than heredity, such as viruses, a high-fat diet, some drugs, radiation, or by-products of our own metabolism called free radicals can cause a mutation. These, in fact, more commonly do the damage. This is why most cancer occurs in people without a hereditary predisposition such as Claudia had. But inheriting the damage puts a person one step closer to cancer than incurring the damage from an environmental factor.

I also told her that the progression from a normal cell to a cancer cell involves mutations to many genes over several years, a whole series of biochemical switches that must be flicked before a cell breaks free of all control and begins to grow wildly.

In the case of the tumor suppressor genes, it is a switch that is turned *off*. But because of a whole other class of genes called oncogenes which, when mutated, cause a switch to turn *on* in order to stimulate unnatural cell growth, scientists are gaining strong clues about how to detect cancer extremely early. Although cancer appears to be cellular anarchy, there is a precise method to its madness. The mutations occur in a definite sequence. So, knowing whether there has been a mutation in an oncogene or in the p53 (sometimes called an antioncogene) will help physicians pin down the precise stage in cancer development a patient has reached.

These changes will be detected by simple tests that will be available by 1997. If a mutation has been hereditary, it will be in all the cells of the body and easily seen in a blood test. But if the mutation has been acquired because of some environmental insult, it may only be in the breast tissue, and a tiny needle biopsy will be done to detect it. In some cases—for both breast and other cancers—even if the mutation was environmentally induced, the changed gene will put out surrogate products that can be detected in the blood. Where physicians look will be, in part, dictated by family history. And, once the detective work is done, molecular therapy—efficient and remarkably lifesaving—will begin.

Researchers are already working on ways to subvert the oncogene. Specific molecules are being developed to fit into "abnormal growth factor receptors" (produced by some oncogenes) in order to block them from stealing nutrients from normal cells and stop the growth of the nascent malignant cell at the same time. And a clinical trial has begun of a monoclonal antibody, an immune system product, targeted specifically at the growth protein manufactured by the HER-2 oncogene, often activated in breast cancer. It will be used routinely within five years to stop progression of breast cancer, especially the most aggressive forms.

There is one oncogene that directs the production of an enzyme that allows cancer cells to spread, or metastasize, throughout the body. And there is yet another that directs the formation of new blood vessels—highways that help bring food to the insatiable tumor. Additional drugs in development will either compete with the enzyme necessary for cancer cells to spread or shut down the process whereby the cells form new blood vessels. Clinical trials using each of these approaches will begin by 1993. By 2000 they will be an integral part of treating cancer.

Equally important in genetic intervention will be correcting the loss of the tumor suppressor genes. Eventually, by 2010, it will be possible to actually replace the lost genes, but ten years earlier we will have a therapy that will be almost as effective. A normal p53 gene produces an enzyme that slows cell growth. It is the loss of this enzyme when the gene is damaged that removes the brake. So instead of using drugs to block the dangerous products of oncogenes, physicians will inject a synthetic replica of the growth-retarding enzyme.

Once these therapies are available to intervene at a much earlier stage, the prognosis for breast cancer will be dramatically improved. It will take a few years after their introduction for the statistics to reflect this, but by 2005, there will be a 50 percent increase in cures and by 2010 a 75 percent increase. This will mean that more than nine out of ten women with breast cancer will be cured.

"That's great to hear," said Claudia, "especially for my daughter Stephanie, who's going to be seventeen next week."

"Absolutely," I said. "By the time she's twenty-one, she'll be able to take a blood test to see if she's inherited the genetic predisposition, and if she has, by the time she's about twenty-five, it will be a simple matter to reverse the effects of any mutations she's had. She has nothing to worry about."

I then explained to Claudia that these same molecular therapies might be used to her advantage as well. Although she was statistically at higher risk for having a recurrence, if it did happen, it wouldn't necessarily occur before some of the genetic diagnostic tests and gene-blocking and enhancing drugs were available.

Even if it were to occur in the next year or two—generally a bad sign—knowledge of oncogenes would likely help her with more conventional treatment. Using tools called molecular probes to analyze cancerous breast tissue, researchers have found that the number of copies of an oncogene a cancer produces determines to a great extent how fast the tumor will recur and tells physicians how aggressive they should be with therapy. By attacking the cancer with a heavy dose of chemotherapy followed by a bone marrow transplant (the chemotherapy would destroy the bone marrow), the results could be improved dramatically.

This approach has already been proven highly successful with neuroblastoma, a rare childhood tumor with a dismal five-year survival rate of only 1 percent. After only two years of using oncogene copies as markers for aggressive treatment, the survival rate went up to a remarkable 40 percent. Since breast cancer figures are not as gloomy to start, the increment of improvement won't be as high, but many more lives will be saved.

Then I talked to Claudia about screening tests. Her doctors had told her to continue monthly self-examination and to have a mammogram every year. I told her that within the next three or four years, another test would be introduced that not only would allow any recurrence to be picked up much earlier than breast examination or mammography but would change the way the cancer would be treated as well.

It is now well known that most breast cancer begins in the ducts, which aren't just conduits to bring milk to the nipple. The ducts are lined by cells that are areas of active metabolism. Instead of waiting to detect an already-developed albeit small tumor on a mammogram, by inserting a tiny needle and withdrawing some tissue from one of the ducts her physician would be able to pick up premalignant changes in the cells before they were ever able to gain a foothold as a tumor, somewhat similar to what is done in a Pap smear.

Then, a procedure would be done that is even more minimal than a lumpectomy. Just the affected duct would be removed, an operation that would leave the tiniest of scars and no disfigurement at all. Shortly thereafter, by 1997 or 1998, even the ductal removal will be unnecessary. Using a laser or an injected solution of "ductal Draino," the cells gone astray will be destroyed without any surgery at all.

By 1999, the procedure will be modified to work at an even earlier stage. Instead of looking for early anatomical changes in the breast cells, physicians, using a syringe, will withdraw some of the fluid from the breast ducts and analyze the microchemical content of it, especially the concentration of calcium. Since the amounts of calcium and other chemicals in the duct fluid may be factors that influence gene mutations, finding an abnormal concentration will allow a doctor to inject a solution that changes the milieu of the cells and reduces the risk of gene transformation.

Although Claudia realized she was still at high risk, the prospects for the future were so bright she knew the odds had just been tipped heavily in her favor.

## SKIN CANCER:
## —————— NEW TECHNOLOGY LEADS THE WAY ——————

In the eighties, we all learned to stop being sun worshippers, or at least unprotected sun worshippers. Now, those of us concerned about skin cancer and premature aging of our skin never venture into the sun without first applying a protective sunscreen. And our worry is increasing, with all the recent publicity about holes in the ozone layer making us even more vulnerable to the damaging effects of ultraviolet rays.

Consequently, sunscreens are improving. The new superpotent varieties not only are more powerful but provide better protection across the board against both types of ultraviolet light: ultraviolet A, or UVA, associated primarily with premature skin aging, and ultraviolet B, or UVB, associated with skin cancer.

Sunscreens are going to remain an important weapon against skin cancer, but they are going to change significantly in the nineties and beyond. And even more important, molecular biology is going to provide us with much better tools to protect us from skin cancer and with a far more effective means of reversing cellular damage that we may have inflicted on ourselves as reckless teenagers.

The watchword of sun protection in the next decade is going to be internal skin-care. Scientists will take a lesson from the ways in which chameleons, frogs and several other creatures react to color changes in their environment, reactions that they are finding extends into the ultraviolet range. This will be sorted out by 1994 when amphibian skin chemistry will be put to work for us. We will have a photosensitive chemical in pill form that will circulate harmlessly in our bodies. When it crosses the skin capillaries, it will react with ultraviolet light that hits the skin. The radiation will change the chemical into something that both binds to our skin cells and absorbs ultraviolet light, protecting our skin cells from any damage. The more exposed and sensitive regions of the skin will build up the highest concentrations of the protective chemical. And a nice cosmetic feature of these pills will be that, besides absorbing ultraviolet rays and protecting our skin, when they bind to the cells they will also confer a tan, one much more natural than the topical products now being sold.

The internal sunscreens will, of course, be more convenient to use than today's creams and lotions, and since they will provide more of a chemical barrier at the site of the potential damage, they will be more effective. But just as is the case with their topical counterparts, they won't be able to protect us against all the cancer-causing damage to the DNA in our skin cells.

By 2000, however, there will be a way to reverse this damage and dramatically reduce our chances for skin cancer. Dermatological researchers are working on DNA repair enzymes that can be topically delivered to skin cells. Once there, these enzymes will restore the DNA to its original state.

## STOPPING DEADLY MELANOMA: A SOLUTION MORE THAN SKIN DEEP

The skin cancer that these approaches are going to be most helpful against are the more common and less dangerous forms: basal cell carcinoma and squamous cell carcinoma. While they both have the capacity to invade the tissues that surround them and to occasionally metastasize throughout the rest of the body, these are rare occurrences, almost nonexistent for basal cell cancer.

In sharp contrast is the other type of skin cancer, malignant melanoma. Although it is completely curable if caught early enough (which theoretically can be said of any cancer), its aggressive nature and its ability to sometimes camouflage itself as a harmless mole often allow it to escape undetected until it's too late, until it has spread throughout the body, something for which melanomas are well known. Add to that the fact that it is the fastest rising cancer in the world, and we have what some dermatologists have called a real epidemic.

Although not as well documented, there is a correlation between sun exposure and the incidence of melanoma, so the same things that will protect against the less virulent skin cancers will help against melanoma, too. But there are several other unknown factors that contribute to melanoma, so scientists are going to have to dig a little deeper to solve the problem. Already they are discovering a mother lode of possibilities in the immune system, which are going to spell both successful treatment and prevention of malignant melanoma.

All cancer cells produce unique proteins on their surface called antigens. These antigens, being foreign substances, should stimulate our immune system to produce antibodies that then bind to and destroy or eliminate the cancer cells. And the T-lymphocytes should be able to mobilize their impressive array of tumor-fighting substances called cytokines—proteins such as interferon, interleukin, tumor necrosis factor and a whole host of other immune-enhancing factors. This does occur automatically to some extent, but the wily cancer cells often resist detection by the immune surveillance system, and antibodies either never get made or don't stick very well to the cancer cells. For years, researchers have been looking for ways to outsmart the cancer cells, to give the immune system a technological boost and make its job easier.

Malignant melanoma has provided the most fertile field for this type of study, and the results we are about to see reflect it. More than with most other types of cancer, our body attempts to mount an immune response against melanoma. Too often, however, it is an ineffectual attack. So this has been a good place to start applying ingenuity.

The process began several years ago, in 1985, when Dr. Steven Rosenberg and his colleagues at the National Cancer Institute developed an imaginative treatment for a large group of terminal cancer patients, including several with metastatic malignant melanoma. Using a special filtration technique, lymphocytes that had been attracted to the tumor but had been unable to mount an effective immune response against it were isolated. These so-called tumor-infiltrating lymphocytes, or TIL—willing of spirit but weak of substance—were then strengthened in the laboratory by incubating them with the immune-enhancing substance interleukin-2. This mixture created a new kind of powerful-sounding cell, dubbed lymphokine-activated killer cells or LAK cells. The LAK cells were then reinfused into the patients, either by themselves or with more interleukin-2.

Considering that every one of these patients had been declared terminal, the 20 percent survival rate obtained couldn't be considered anything but a resounding success, loudly trumpeted (and exaggerated) by the media, to the point where the switchboards at the National Cancer Institute were hopelessly jammed for days, while people unsuccessfully tried to get themselves on the still-experimental therapy.

The next step occurred in 1990, when Dr. Rosenberg provided considerably more muscle to the immunological treatment of terminal malignant melanoma patients, launching the first genetic therapy of cancer. Once again, tumor-infiltrating lymphocytes were isolated from melanoma patients. Then, in the laboratory, instead of merely incubating them with an immune-enhancing substance as had been done earlier, a new gene was introduced to the patient's tumor-infiltrating lymphocytes, a gene for the cancer-killing substance known as tumor necrosis factor. This gave these genetically engineered cells the power to make the tumor necrosis factor themselves, which they began to do after they were returned to the patients with melanoma. Although it will be 1993 before definitive results are in, early figures on remissions look very encouraging.

Within a year of that, there will be an even further refinement. This time, the middleman lymphocytes will be eliminated. The gene for the tumor necrosis factor will be inserted directly into the melanoma cells, thereby planting within them the seeds of their own destruction. When this gene starts pumping out tumor necrosis factor, the substance will promptly kill the cells that made it.

At first, this will be performed the way other genetic therapy is now being done, by removing the cells and adding the destructive gene. But within ten years the process will reach the ultimate in elegance and simplicity. Using immunological homing techniques such as monoclonal antibodies, the laboratory step will be eliminated. Attached to these antibodies will be the gene for tumor necrosis factor, and when injected, they will deliver it specifically and only to the melanoma cells. The "designer cancer cells" will be created right in the patient.

This sort of genetic engineering of the immune system will play a major role in the future treatment of advanced cases of malignant melanoma and, with different combinations of immune cells and immune-enhancing cytokine proteins, of other types of cancer as well. That is when we will see a truly remarkable increase in cures from this deadly disease.

The immune system is so complex it makes sense that there is more than one way to accomplish the same goal. Dr. M. Rigdon

Lentz, an oncologist in the desert of Indio, California, is trying a different approach to the treatment of terminal cancer, with especially good results in melanoma.

One of the problems that has perplexed immunologists through the years has been the protected status of the fetus developing in the mother's womb. Since genes are inherited from both parents, and since there is a luxurious exchange of blood between mother and fetus, it is certain that the mother is exposed to some proteins that her immune system should recognize as foreign. Just as if the fetus were an organ transplanted from an incompatible donor, the immune system should mount an all-out attack on the fetus and reject it. But it doesn't, and studying the reason why has led Dr. Lentz to a unique form of immunotherapy for cancer.

He found that the fetus produces a small molecular weight inhibitory substance which protects it from being recognized by the policemen of the mother's immune system. Using an ultrafiltration system to specifically remove this substance from the blood of pregnant goats, he was immediately and repeatedly able to induce abortions.

Dr. Lentz then found that cancer cells produce the same kind of molecular inhibitory substance which helps them evade the immune detection system. Once this factor was removed by ultrafiltration, the power of the immune system was unleashed against the cancers. Tumors shrank in incredibly short times. In a couple of dramatic cases, melanomas literally "fell off patients in the bed," Dr. Lentz told me.

This, though, is still experimental therapy, and not yet FDA approved. The major bug in the system is a serious problem with having tumors destroyed too rapidly, something called tumor lysis syndrome, which actually killed a few patients. On the positive side, though, autopsies showed that the tumors of these otherwise unfortunate patients had completely disappeared, and couldn't be detected even under the microscope. Although this is truly a case of "the operation being successful and the patient dying," this form of immunotherapy is going to be an impressive addition to the arsenal against melanoma and other terminal forms of cancer.

Far better than having to devise ingenious methods to treat metastatic melanoma would be to use the power of the immune system to prevent it from occurring in the first place. The best way of doing this is turning out to be an anticancer vaccine.

Imagine, just as is now done for viral diseases such as measles and mumps, going to your doctor and having an inoculation that will protect you against the development of cancer in the future. This has long been a dream of both oncologists and immunologists. Even in the sixties when I was a graduate student in immunology, I remember researchers in our department working on this problem. Tumor cells, though, are complicated, and it turned out to be no small feat to isolate their distinguishing proteins which, when injected, would stimulate the production of not only antibodies against the cancer cells, but ones that would destroy them.

But buoyed by advances in molecular biology, scientists have been able to amplify the surface proteins on melanoma cells and recently have isolated a melanoma gene. Both of these achievements have given the melanoma vaccine a feeling of reality. After many years and many false starts, we can see that this will soon be possible. Within five years, following surgical removal of a melanoma, patients will receive a vaccine to prevent a recurrence, and within ten years, this approach will be used to prevent melanomas in healthy people.

The most promising approach so far is one being taken by researchers at Mt. Sinai Medical Center in Miami, Florida, and at the German Cancer Research Center in Heidelberg, an elegant blend of traditional and high-tech immunology. Using a vaccinia virus—the same harmless virus used more than one hundred years ago by immunology pioneer Edward Jenner to protect milkmaids against smallpox—they have "tricked" the immune system into making potent antibodies against malignant melanoma. The virus is introduced into the melanoma cells, and these newly created hybrid cells express both viral proteins and melanoma proteins on their surface. Since our immune systems are already well versed in making antibodies against the vaccinia virus, these cells are like waving a red flag to the antibody-producing cells. They make antibodies against both the virus and the melanoma proteins, far better antimelanoma antibodies than would be made against the evasive melanoma cells alone.

This was first tested in the late 1980s against patients who had melanoma that had spread to their lymph nodes, patients at high risk for a postsurgical recurrence. Astonishingly, 80 percent survived for two years without recurrence. It is now being evaluated in a large multicenter study of more than two hundred patients. After some modifications in the vaccine to make it even more effective, we will see this used on melanoma patients after surgery in 1995.

An even more sophisticated approach is going to involve genetic engineering. Rather than mixing melanoma and vaccinia virus cells together, researchers at the National Cancer Institute are taking advantage of the recent isolation of the gene in melanoma cells that is responsible for making the proteins the immune system can recognize as foreign. Inserting this gene into the harmless vaccinia virus will create a cell that, when inoculated into patients, can continually manufacture viral proteins to attract both the immune system and melanoma proteins, making sure that enough antibodies get made. By 2000, this method is going to be used not only to prevent recurrences but to protect high-risk patients (for example those who are fair-skinned and who spend a lot of time in the sun) from ever developing melanoma.

Since the proteins produced by cancer cells are all different, there won't ever be just one anticancer vaccine. But we can foresee the day when a series of injections will protect us against most cancers.

## LUNG CANCER IS ON THE WAY OUT

As we age, even if we don't smoke, the pink, resilient lungs we are born with are changed into gray, carbon-flecked ones that are somewhat less compliant. These are marked changes but nothing compared with what the lungs of a lung cancer victim look like. Although I performed more than two hundred autopsies as a first-year resident in pathology more than fifteen years ago, I still vividly recall my first case of lung cancer.

As I cut into those lungs, my first thought was that it resembled an alien invasion. The beautiful and delicate intricacies of the respiratory tract had been almost entirely replaced by spreading white, rock-hard tissue that had choked off the bronchial passages. When I sectioned the liver, metastatic nodules of the same tissue defiantly studded the surface.

This person had been a smoker, as are 90 percent of the 143,000 Americans who will die of lung cancer this year. And, of course, the single most important thing that we can do to reduce our chances of getting lung cancer is to not smoke. Thanks to some aggressive public education we are inching our way toward the smokeless society that former surgeon general Koop foresaw. It's going to be some time before we achieve it, though, probably about twenty years, and not till the genetics of addiction are worked out better so the appropriate smoking substitutes can be developed.

But, although almost all cases of lung cancer occur in smokers, the converse is not true. Most smokers don't get lung cancer—only about one in eight. We all can cite an example of a relative or someone else we knew who smoked two packs of Turkish cigarettes a day for sixty years and died of natural causes at ninety-four. So there must be something else besides just smoking involved. The answer, as is going to be the answer to so many medical problems in the next couple of decades, is being provided with genetics and molecular biology. When everything is worked out, not only will physicians be in a far better position to treat and prevent lung cancer, but—and I never thought I'd say this—they may actually tell some patients it's all right to smoke!

Just as with breast cancer and most other cancers, a small percentage of cases of lung cancer are inherited, but studying them provides important molecular clues to the development of the vast majority of cancers that aren't hereditary. In 1991, researchers at the National Cancer Institute determined the familial pattern to be the result of a mutation in just one gene.

Smokers who had inherited this particular mutant gene were more than six times as likely to have lung cancer by the age of sixty as smokers who hadn't inherited the mutant gene. But nonsmokers who inherited the mutant gene weren't at any greater risk of developing lung cancer than other nonsmokers. Clearly smoking is still involved, but how?

Further research showed that this familial gene directs the production of an enzyme that accelerates the activation of the cancer-causing chemicals in cigarette smoke. There are so many of these chemicals in smoke that even without the activating enzyme it is still possible to eventually develop lung cancer, but it is much less likely. And since nonsmokers with the mutant gene are not exposed to the cancer-causing chemicals, producing the enzyme doesn't increase their risk.

Just the knowledge of this one mutant gene is going to improve lung cancer detection and treatment, and individualize it. Within a year, by 1993, there will be a simple blood test available that will be able to detect the presence of the mutant gene. Although at that stage physicians are still going to be telling all their patients not to smoke, someone who has this mutant gene will be warned even more strongly that he or she is risking a life.

If attempts to convince these smokers to quit are unsuccessful, they will be subjected to regular screening tests, not chest x-rays, because by the time it is detected that way the cancer is often inoperable, but sputum samples, to look for the presence of abnormal cells before they have coalesced into a tumor. Collecting a workable sputum sample often has to be done by bronchoscopy— a procedure in which a tube is inserted deep into the respiratory tract. This is a moderately invasive and expensive procedure, so it isn't feasible to use as a screening test on everyone, even on all smokers. But it will be useful for the highest-risk smokers who inherited the abnormal gene, and will significantly improve their prognosis. Using lasers and localized microsurgery, the focus of abnormal cells will be removed.

Just as with other cancers, though, inheriting this one mutant gene isn't a *sine qua non* for developing lung cancer. Scientists have estimated that somewhere between five and ten genes have to be mutated before cancer develops. Cigarette smoke is the main environmental factor responsible for flicking the biochemical switches. That's why smokers who don't inherit the enzyme-activating gene are still at far higher risk of developing lung cancer than nonsmokers. Over the years, substances in cigarette smoke can activate and deactivate the whole series of genes that eventually result in cancer.

For some reason, though, most smokers escape this damage to their genes and avoid lung cancer. It may be that there are other hereditary mutations which those predisposed to lung cancer inherit. There may be other unrecognized environmental factors besides cigarette smoke that damage normal genes. Undoubtedly, the molecular basis by which most smokers escape lung cancer will be determined within the next ten years. But we won't have to wait that long before valuable, lifesaving information can be given to smokers.

What is being worked on—available by 1998—is an understanding of all the genes that must be mutated before lung cancer develops. Shortly thereafter, there will be blood tests and tests on cells secreted into the sputum to determine what, if any, genetic mutations have taken place. For smokers, this will be part of their routine physical exam. The knowledge of which genes do what will be so widespread that, on the basis of this test, a physician will be able to tell his patient how far along he is down the lung cancer road, and precisely what are the chances of developing it. If there are no mutations, or if the mutations are at an early stage in the malignancy sequence, a smoker may decide to continue, and without much risk of developing lung cancer.

In addition, there will be molecular intervention therapies that will rehabilitate criminal genes by either blocking the dangerous substances they produce or providing the beneficial ones they have stopped making. All of this will dramatically reduce the risk of lung cancer in those who choose to continue smoking. Of course, there will still be heart disease, emphysema and other smoking-related illnesses to contend with, but it is likely that molecular detection and protection mechanisms will be developed for related diseases as well.

Detecting early molecular damage to genes in the respiratory tree, and instituting remedial therapies at just the right time, is going to revolutionize our approach to lung cancer. But there is another tack researchers are taking that will yield results even sooner.

It involves, not detecting whether a gene has been mutated by cigarette smoke, but determining *how* the smoke does this so we can prevent it from happening. Although there are a variety of carcinogenic substances in cigarette smoke, the most notorious are free radicals, promiscuously reactive chemicals which populate cigarette smoke like rush hour in New Delhi.

As Dr. Peter Cerutti, Director of Carcinogenesis at the Swiss Cancer Institute in Lausanne, explained to me, free radicals are very capable of mutating genes, activating oncogenes and deactivating tumor suppressor genes. There are, though, substances that can protect us from the damaging effects of the free radicals in cigarette smoke. Known as antioxidants (because the chemical reaction that free radicals induce is oxidation), they are represented by vitamins E and C, the vitamin A precursor beta-carotene and the trace mineral selenium. Several epidemiological studies have shown that higher levels of vitamin E and beta-carotene in the bloodstream are associated with a lower risk of lung cancer among smokers. Studies of this kind prompted the National Cancer Institute to invest more than one hundred million dollars in the mid-

1980s to see if taking supplements of these antioxidant vitamins would prevent the development of cancer.

The most publicized of these studies, in which more than twenty thousand American physicians have been taking either beta-carotene or a placebo for several years while being periodically examined for the incidence of all cancer, is due to be completed by 1993. Added to previous studies, this one and several others will almost certainly demonstrate a protective effect of beta-carotene and other antioxidants. And it will begin a new era of mainstream medicine: chemoprevention. Since free radicals are produced by many other things besides cigarette smoke—drugs, radiation, viruses, our own metabolism—doctors will begin to routinely advise all their patients, smokers and nonsmokers, to take supplements of antioxidants such as vitamin E, selenium and beta-carotene, and by 1994 other carotenoids (relatives of beta-carotene) will be found to be even more effective. The best candidate is a substance called lycopene, found in abundance in tomatoes.

To add to these natural antioxidants there will be new classes of antioxidants generated by computer programs that will specifically isolate the portion of the antioxidant molecule that protects the genes and are side-effect free. These novel antioxidants will be even better at preventing mutations than most of the natural substances.

Scientists are also finding two additional points that are going to be used routinely by our doctors. First, not everyone responds to antioxidants in the same way. Some people, most smokers for example, need to take more to achieve the same protective level. Second, the antioxidant defense system in our body is multitiered, that is, the antioxidants are dependent on each other. Therefore, as part of our routine physicals within three or four years, physicians will take a blood sample and measure our antioxidant profile. If we are below an optimal protective level in one or more antioxidants, we will be advised to take particular supplements (smokers will take the most powerful synthetic antioxidants because they will be at higher risk of genetic damage) and have the profile repeated some months later. Thereafter, it will be regularly measured to make sure it stays in the optimal protective range.

## —— TAKING THE WORRY OUT OF PROSTATE CANCER ——

If you are a man, considering no other factors, there is a one in ten chance that you will develop prostate cancer. It is the most common malignancy in men. Those are still pretty good odds, but not so long that most men don't sometimes worry about getting the disease. And as we age, or if we have a family history, the chances increase significantly. A large familial study at Johns Hopkins University Medical School recently concluded that if your father or brother had prostate cancer, your chances of acquiring it are doubled. If your grandfather or uncle also had prostate cancer, your chances are nine times greater! But if you are a middle-aged man in one of these categories, you aren't going to have to worry about these sobering statistics much longer.

Just as is the case for all other cancers, prostate cancer is ultimately a genetic disease, the loss of cellular control over growth. Scientists have not yet identified which genes, when changed, eventually result in prostate cancer, but using the same molecular probing techniques that are being applied to the investigation of other cancers, there is no doubt that the complex genetics of prostate cancer will be unraveled, most certainly within the next ten years, probably even sooner. The advances in genetics, immunology, laboratory cell culture and new noninvasive imaging techniques are going to make it possible to detect virtually every case of prostate cancer at an early stage, when it is still curable. And in most cases the cure won't have to be surgery. There will be not only new blood tests for hereditary predispositions, but tests on prostate tissue samples for acquired changes in the genes as men age. And, of course, within five years after that, there will be molecular therapies to counteract these genetic mutations.

Within twenty years even most of these innovative techniques will become unnecessary. There will be introduced instead a novel preventive methodology, one that will be considered strange and be opposed as too unnatural by segments in both the medical and nonmedical community, but which will wipe out any possibility of developing prostate cancer.

In 1991, we got a glimpse of the future when a study on more than two thousand men found that a simple blood test could provide an effective, widespread method of screening for prostate cancer. The test was more accurate than the standard rectal exam recommended to all men over forty, increasing the chances of detecting prostate cancer by 20 percent. But it is still far from infallible at its present stage of development. And until the accuracy of the test is improved, physicians will use it in conjunction with a rectal exam.

That will change within the next ten years, though. The blood test that is currently being used measures a particular protein produced by the prostate, called prostate-specific antigen or PSA. Before being demonstrated of value in screening early cases of prostate cancer, it had been used for several years to assess treatment and progression of known cases. PSA is only one of many specific antigens that the prostate gland produces. New monoclonal antibody techniques are being developed that will be able to target even more revealing prostate proteins and diagnose cancer far earlier and more accurately. By the end of this decade, we will see blood tests used that are so precise they will be the only diagnostic method needed.

Antigen-detection techniques won't be the only interim confirmatory tests used to diagnose prostate cancer. When a patient has a positive blood test, his physician will sometimes perform a prostatic massage, a moderately uncomfortable procedure but one that will yield important results. The cells harvested by this massage will be grown in the laboratory, in a medium that limits the survival of normal cells but allows tumor cells to grow and multiply. After just a week in the cell culture, it will be known whether there is prostate cancer.

If caught early enough, surgery for prostate cancer is often curative, but it is not minor surgery and there are often serious residual effects, including incontinence and impotence. The new diagnostic tests, though, are going to be able to detect cancer so early that physicians will easily and successfully implement a nonsurgical treatment.

This is coming, and it is coming relatively soon. A whole class of drugs called 5-alpha-reductase inhibitors are already being introduced for the nonsurgical shrinkage of benign prostatic hyperplasia, or BPH, the noncancerous enlargement that affects all men as they age. Although the basic mechanisms by which cancer and benign enlargement of the prostate occur are different, both are widely believed to be stimulated by male hormones. Since the new drugs inhibit this hormonal effect (without any loss of libido) there is optimism that they, or derivatives of them, will be useful for the early treatment of prostate cancer as well as benign enlargement. Within ten years, biochemistry is going to be added to, and may eventually replace, surgery as the primary therapy for prostate cancer.

Everything we've talked about till now is going to remarkably reduce the incidence of prostate cancer and deaths from it, but in reality there is really only one surefire, 100 percent guaranteed way of avoiding prostate cancer: not having a prostate.

As bizarre as this might appear, it very likely will be the ultimate intervention fifteen years from now. Unlike other organs in our body, the prostate has a usefulness that we outlive. Its main function is to contribute lubricating substances to the semen, so when a man's reproductive (not his sexual) life is complete, the prostate becomes a "disposable organ," just sitting there growing larger and waiting to develop cancer. Why not remove it?

Subjecting men to prophylactic surgery after they pass the age when fathering a child is desirable is unreasonable in view of potential operative complications. But how about eliminating the prostate another way?

The answer is going to be provided by immunology. Variants of the same monoclonal antibodies that will be used to precisely diagnose early prostate cancer will be used to destroy the outdated gland. Tagged onto specific monoclonal antibodies will be a cocktail of several toxic drugs, multiple warheads aimed at one target: the prostate. After a series of injections, the gland will quietly wither away and pose no threat.

At first, this technique will be used only in those with a high genetic risk for prostate cancer, but twenty years from now it will become a routine part of passage into later middle age and beyond.

## COLON CANCER:
## —— MOLECULAR DIAGNOSTICS AND TREATMENT ——

We are coming so close to understanding just how some types of cancer are caused that the anticipation and excitement in the scientific community are palpable. Colon cancer, one of the leading killers, is the cancer on which the most work has been done.

Dr. Bert Vogelstein and his colleagues at the Johns Hopkins Oncology Center in Baltimore have almost completely worked out the genetic sequence of events in colon cancer from normal cell, to benign tumor, to premalignant tumor, to localized malignant tumor, to metastatic tumor.

We are only a year or two away from being able to have routine molecular diagnostic tests performed to see if we have had any genetic damage in our colon. Not only will such tests be far easier and cheaper to perform than testing the stool for occult blood followed by sigmoidoscopy, but the results are going to drastically change the incidence and the prognosis of colon cancer. In twenty years, we will wipe out more than 90 percent of it.

For a diagnosis we will require the same stool sample. Molecular probes will search the colonic cells within the sample for the presence of either an activation in a cancer-enhancing gene or a deactivation in a cancer-suppressing gene. No molecular diagnosis could possibly be earlier. And because the sequence for colon cancer development is being determined so precisely, the results of the stool analysis will provide information about not only whether the cells are perfectly normal but, if there has been a mutation, where in the sequence the mutation is.

Once the mutations in colon genes have been detected, perfectly tailored molecular therapies will be given to break the chain of events. Just as with breast cancer, in the case of the growth-enhancing oncogenes the therapy will block them, or if the damage has been the loss of a tumor suppressor gene, the therapy will provide the necessary growth-retarding product. These therapies will be available by 1998.

Beyond this, under development is the ultimate molecular treatment of colon cancer: rehabilitating the incipient cancer cell rather than executing it, supplying a new gene rather than altering gene products. The notorious p53 gene we mentioned earlier in connection with breast cancer is also being demonstrated to be involved in other cancers, especially colon cancer. In this case, it may be one of the final mutations necessary before a benign cell turns into a malignant one.

The same group of scientists at Johns Hopkins also demonstrated that it is possible to shut down the cancer engine once it has been turned on. Using colon cancer cells growing in a test tube, in which molecular analysis had shown damaged copies of the tumor suppressor p53 gene, they added a normal copy of the gene and, incredibly, were able to stop the cancer cells from growing. This finding has tremendous significance to the future treatment of cancer. The braking ability supplied by the p53 is so important that even after the cells have already turned malignant, adding the p53 gene can stop them from growing any further. The engine may not be reversible, but this experiment shows that it can be stopped.

Once this is available for use with patients, even if someone fails to have a molecular detection test early enough to avoid the development of a tumor, supplying the p53 gene will be able to cure them completely. But this approach won't be available until 2005. The trick will be to get the normal copy of the tumor suppressor gene into just those cells that are missing it. Injecting it indiscriminately would flood normal cells and give them an extra copy of a gene they don't need, with potentially disastrous metabolic consequences. Normal cells would shut down and die.

The scientists working today are performing miracles, though, and there is no doubt they will accomplish this as well. Before 2010, a copy of the suppressor gene will be linked to a synthetically constructed protein which in turn will be linked to a monoclonal antibody directed specifically to the colon cancer cells (even early in their development, they produce unique proteins). This fusion protein will home in on the cells that need the tumor suppressor gene. The fusion protein will also be made with specific properties so that the young cancer cells engulf the delivered package, a molecular Trojan horse. The developing tumor will be stopped dead in its tracks.

## OTHER CANCERS OF THE GASTROINTESTINAL TRACT: — UNCOMMON AND DEADLY, BUT NOT FOR LONG —

Colon cancer is by far the most common malignancy of the gastrointestinal tract, so it makes sense that more human and financial resources have been devoted to deciphering its modus operandi. But the tract is a long tube from mouth to anus, and every inch of it can be ravaged by cancer. And even though they aren't part of the digestive tube, the liver, gallbladder and pancreas make vital contributions to digestion, so they are often included as part of the tract as well.

In developed countries, gastrointestinal cancers are rare and usually devastating when they do occur. In other parts of the world, they are equally devastating but much more common. Liver cancer, for example, is uncommon in the United States but, because it is the leading cancer in Africa, ranks number five on the global scale.

And most of the African victims are young people, in their early thirties.

For most of these gastrointestinal cancers, the main problem is lack of early detection. There are no readily accessible cells that shed in fluids such as sputum, urine or stool. And it isn't easy enough or safe enough to routinely insert tiny needles to remove tissue samples from the pancreas or liver, such as will be done for screening early breast cancer.

The approach in the future is going to begin with a universal test, followed by more focused detective work if necessary. This will be provided before 2000 by a cheap monoclonal antibody test.

Because the genes that turn them on produce some abnormal proteins, every cancer tips its hand early, as long as we are looking. By developing a series of monoclonal antibodies that will detect unusual products in the blood, but not necessarily where these products came from, physicians will get an idea that a young cancer is brewing. Then more sophisticated and more targeted diagnostic tests will be done.

First, there will be more refined blood tests, more specific monoclonal antibodies and molecular probes, to try to pin down the organ source of the abnormal gene product. This will then be followed by advanced imaging techniques. In the case of solid organs such as the liver and pancreas, the procedure will be a PET or SPECT scan. These tests do not look for anatomical abnormalities but instead have the ability to detect abnormal areas of metabolism. If any are detected, a tiny tissue biopsy will be taken for molecular and anatomical analysis.

If a cancer is found, it will be treated according to its stage of development. If it is early enough, molecular blocking therapies will be given. If it is a little later, monoclonal antibodies tagged with radioactive substances specific for the liver or pancreas will be used to destroy the tumor. Sometimes, a combination of immune and molecular therapy will be used. In any case, we will see a 75 percent improvement in survival from liver and pancreatic cancer in the next fifteen years.

For liver cancer, there will be some additional help. Some environmental risk factors are known, which have been shown to activate cancer-causing genes. Addressing these in the next ten years is going to make a big difference in prevention. Aflatoxin, a fungal poison which contaminates grain stored improperly in warm, moist places, is a major culprit. So is hepatitis B virus. Under the auspices of the World Health Organization, better food storage and more effective development and widespread use of antihepatitis B virus vaccines are both going to contribute to the decline in liver cancer.

If on the basis of the molecular and immunological markers, cancer of the actual digestive tube is suspected (from the esophagus to the large intestine), PET and SPECT scans will also be done to look for metabolic abnormalities. In addition, a procedure called ultrasonic endoscopy will be employed; a fiberoptic tube will allow the physician to scan up and down the entire digestive tract, looking for abnormal clumps of cells and vaporizing them immediately with an attached laser.

## LEUKEMIAS:
—————— ADULTS CATCH UP WITH CHILDREN ——————

For the past several years, epidemiologists have looked at the cancer survival data through every possible statistical microscope and from every angle imaginable, and yet they still disagree about our progress in the war on cancer. One thing, though, that they do all agree on is that we have made exhilarating strides in treating childhood leukemias, only a blip in the total scheme of cancers, but when children are involved, we don't care about numbers.

The chemotherapy that has proven so successful in the common types of childhood leukemia hasn't worked nearly as well in the adult forms. Some exciting developments are on the horizon, however, advances that will allow the control of the disease in adults as well as in children and will improve childhood leukemia treatment even further.

For the gene-altering reasons we have discussed, cancer cells are like juvenile delinquents, growing and acting wildly while in a difficult stage of development. Some of the molecular approaches being cultivated are an attempt to remove the bad influences on the cell so that it will grow normally. But there is another way being explored to essentially the same end, and it is showing the greatest promise in leukemias.

It is called differentiation therapy, supplying the cell with substances that it lost when the cancer-causing genes took over. Restoring these substances to the cells can put them back on the normal track they were on when they were diverted by cancer.

One of the best examples of this approach was demonstrated in promyelocytic leukemia, a rare type that accounts for only 15 percent of adult leukemias. The differentiation therapy used a substance that at first seems surprising but that will have implications for more common types of leukemia.

Most of us have heard of tretinoin under its trade name Accutane, the vitamin A derivative that has become a cure for acne, and that can reverse some of the skin aging caused by sun exposure. It was a close cousin of Accutane that was able to revert leukemia cells back to normal. In normal development, vitamin A is necessary for differentiation, for pushing cells along the path to become skin cells, or kidney cells, or whatever kind of cells they are supposed to be. In order to do this, the vitamin A must first attach to receptors on the cell surface and then send the appropriate differentiation message.

The leukemia cells, because of a gene mutation, had lost this crucial receptor and couldn't differentiate any further toward normal white blood cells. But they could grow as immature white blood cells and cause leukemia. Enter tretinoin, the powerful vitamin A relative, which was so effective as a differentiating factor that the leukemia cells were convinced to begin to become normal cells, even without the receptor. Strikingly, nine of eleven patients with leukemia went into remission.

By the mid-nineties, other potent vitamin A derivatives, many of which are presently being researched, are going to be used as differentiating factors to treat leukemia. And there are a whole variety of cellular growth and differentiating factors being explored, substances that can send the right signals to cancer cells to make them or at least their progeny normal. By 2001, this is going to be an important mainstay in our successful conquest of all cancer, a success that ten years ago even the most optimistic among us wouldn't have even dreamed of.

# 7

# The End of Coronary Disease

THE REVERSIBILITY OF CORONARY HEART DISEASE EITHER BY changes in lifestyle or by drug therapy is, by now, old news. Yet, as good as this news continues to be, coronary disease is still the number one killer in industrialized societies. But this will soon change. In the next twenty years progress in our battle to end this disease will be breathtaking. It will happen as the result of a symphonic cooperation among cardiologists, cardiovascular surgeons, geneticists, molecular biologists, radiologists and biomedical engineers and will reach a crescendo in 2020, by which time we will have eliminated more than 90 percent of the problem.

To begin with, we've already developed some understanding of exactly how atherosclerosis occurs at the molecular level. Research is still primarily in the laboratory, but before the end of the decade there will be the first clinical applications of these findings to prevention and treatment. Ten years after that, by 2010, molecular prevention and treatment will be virtually the only way of handling coronary disease. Cardiologists and cardiovascular surgeons will move on to becoming sophisticated genetic technicians.

But we have a lot of living to do in the meantime. So let's focus our attention first on the next five or six years, during which we're going to see some remarkable improvements and refinements in the course we've already charted. Between now and the breakthrough years, better ways of measuring and controlling our cholesterol levels and new and far more successful ways of diagnosing and treating existing coronary disease will have a significant impact on the number of lives saved as well as on the quality of life for cardiac patients.

We've been reminded for the past several years to "know our cholesterol number." Many of us have taken the next step and learned the values of our "bad" LDL and "good" HDL cholesterol. This is about to be refined even further. As a prelude to the molecular approaches to come, within the next few years, our doctors will begin to routinely measure new and different subclasses of LDL and HDL cholesterol as well as other classes of the cholesterol-carrying particles, compounds such as IDL (intermediate density lipoprotein), "dense LDL," apoprotein A and B, to name only a few.

The elegant research in the 1970s by University of Texas researchers (and subsequent Nobel laureates) Michael Brown and Joseph Goldstein, who discovered the existence of receptors for LDL cholesterol on the surface of cells, was the beginning of our understanding of the exact nature of fat and cholesterol metabolism in our bodies. Their work opened up a treasure chest of molecular pathways, and it has since become clear that our body's lipid control system is highly complex, involving a number of diverse components. What is also clear is that the functioning of every one of these components is under some form of genetic control, whether it's the structure of the cholesterol-carrying particles themselves, the receptors on their surface or one of many enzymes involved in the process.

Each year, new discoveries are being made in this area of research, and by 2000, the genetics and molecular biology of this system will be figured out completely. When we reach that point, cholesterol and other lipid regulation will become thoroughly individualized. It will be possible to biochemically dissect and control each component of our cholesterol metabolic pathway. And this control is going to bring all of us a welcome and extraordinary benefit, an early risk factor evaluation that will be followed by more aggressive and individual therapy for those in greatest danger of developing a heart attack.

Imagine that your father, sixty-eight years old, has had angina for the past two years, since 1993. Despite all your warnings that he should try to control his cholesterol, exercise regularly and stop smoking, he has stubbornly adhered to his lifestyle of the past thirty years and eventually developed coronary artery disease. Now, with medication no longer effectively stemming his chest pain, his doctor says it is time to assess the degree of blockage in his coronary arteries and, if necessary, do something about it.

If this were happening today, the next step would be to have him check into the hospital for an angiogram. A catheter would be threaded into the femoral artery in his groin and up into the coronary arteries covering the heart. Contrast dye would be injected, and x-ray images would be taken of the blood vessels. Your father would be returned to his room and have to lie perfectly still on his back for several hours. Assuming no complications, he would be discharged the next morning and then have to wait for a call from his physician a few days later with the results. If a blockage was revealed by the angiogram, the therapy would most likely be angioplasty. Under local anesthesia, a catheter containing a balloon would be threaded up from his groin into his coronary artery. When the point of obstruction was reached, the balloon would be inflated, squashing the plaque against the side of the artery wall and re-opening circulation. All in all, not a horrible experience, certainly better than having to undergo coronary bypass surgery. But it could, and will, be improved by 1995. Instead of having to be hospitalized, your father would go as an outpatient for a procedure that would determine the extent of blockage in his arteries in an entirely safe and noninvasive way. He would be totally awake and alert throughout the diagnostic test, and not even a local anesthetic would be used, as is necessary for an angiogram.

The technique employed is called a coronary MRI. In the past few years, we've heard quite a bit about MRI, or magnetic resonance imaging, a safe, noninvasive diagnostic technique based on the characteristic absorption of energy by different tissues when placed in a magnetic field. It is being used for a variety of diagnostic procedures, from the detection of brain tumors to examining sore shoulders in athletes. But MRI has not been applicable to outlining the coronary arteries because it hasn't been "fast enough" to capture the subtle movements of blood in the coronary vessels. The invasive angiogram has remained the standard diagnostic technique.

Fast MRI, though, is just about here, and certainly will be sophisticated enough by 1995, so that it will be a simple matter to lie in the MRI tube for just a few minutes, receive no radiation and come out at the other end along with a perfect picture of the circulation in the coronary arteries.

If, for example, your father is again the patient, after the coronary MRI is performed, the cardiologist and radiologist study the clear images of his coronary arteries and, just as his symptoms suggested, find that he has significant blockage in two of the three main vessels. The coronary MRI is so detailed that it also shows the blockages are not the same in each of the arteries, information that will affect how they are treated. In the left main coronary artery, there is a small area of total occlusion, which looks recent and which probably accounts for the recent escalation in severity of symptoms. This is followed by an elongated, calcified area of narrowing, or stenosis, a condition that has almost certainly been building up over the years. In the right coronary artery, there is only stenosis, with no area of complete occlusion.

After consulting with each other, the cardiovascular surgeon and the cardiologist meet with you and your father in their office adjoining the MRI room. They explain that your father indeed has significant coronary artery disease that can and should be treated surgically. When your father looks worried, they further explain that he will not need a bypass, nor will he even have to check into the hospital to have an angioplasty. The procedure can be done right now, right here, and he will be able to go home within three hours.

A nurse comes into the office and takes your father into a large, gleaming theater called the Endovascular Intervention Suite. The room is full of state-of-the-art high-tech equipment, including an array of television monitors mounted on the ceiling, video recorders, a robotic video camera, complex-looking computers, and a series of unusual-appearing instruments. Unlike other operating theaters, the table is nonmetallic, giving the place a soft edge. Indeed, even though the nurses, technicians and the cardiovascular surgeon are dressed in traditional operating room garb, and the whole suite is decidedly space-age, there is an aura of friendliness, of confidence, of noninvasiveness about what is going to happen.

The doctor explains to your father that for this procedure he will need an anesthetic, but it will be only a mild one and he will be able to remain awake for the entire ninety minutes that the surgery will take. She shows you the observation dome, from which you are welcome to watch in person, but you choose to go to a side suite and observe everything clearly on a television monitor.

The nurse starts an IV and begins to infuse the mild anesthetic. Ten minutes later, the surgeon makes a small incision on the underside of your father's left arm and inserts a thin, unusual-looking catheter with several small, elaborate attachments on the tip. The nurse watching with you on the monitor explains that this is a laser catheter, the energy being delivered by a fiberoptic system, a technical advance that makes the lasers much more efficient. She further explains that the type of laser being used is also unique. It is called a holmium laser and is very different from the lasers that were studied in the late 1980s and early 1990s. Those lasers were so-called hot-tipped, and numerous reports indicated that they were quite inefficient. Not only did the heat from them injure the lining of the blood vessel, but they weren't very good at removing tissue. For both of these reasons, the rate at which the treated coronary arteries closed up again was still about an unacceptable 40 percent, no better than the complication rate with the balloon angioplasty, its main drawback.

The holmium laser, on the other hand, is called a "cool" laser. The energy from the fiberoptic system is delivered in the mid-infrared range and inflicts much less thermal damage to the artery wall. The reocclusion rate has been less than 10 percent and would soon be even better than that. In addition, the holmium laser is able to remove much more unwanted tissue than its hot predecessors, and as an additional benefit, it's even cheaper than the older models.

The nurse shows you on the monitor that the tip of the laser catheter has reached your father's coronary arteries. Watching the monitor herself, the surgeon guides the laser into the left coronary artery, the one that the MRI had shown to have a one-half-centimeter area of complete occlusion just after the origin of the artery. Although the collateral arteries are still able to bring enough blood to the heart muscle normally supplied by the left coronary artery to avoid a full-blown heart attack, this is the main reason for your father's chest pain, and if this occlusion is not opened soon, it very likely would result in a heart attack within the next few months.

When the monitor shows that the tip of the laser has reached the area of occlusion, the surgeon activates a burst of energy that blasts its way through the completely occluded area. Next, she stops to check her work so far. Mounted on the end of the catheter, along with the holmium laser, is a tiny camera called an angioscope, activated with the same fiberoptic energy used for the laser. When the surgeon turns on the camera with a remote control switch, an image of the interior of the artery is projected onto the monitor. Success! There is a smooth, round hole, or lumen, through the center of the previously occluded segment of the artery. The picture is so sharp, and magnified so much on the television monitor, you get the feeling you are actually inside the artery.

The physician stops for a moment and asks your father how he is feeling. Your father says he feels perfectly well, as if nothing is happening. Then the surgeon turns on the speaker in your monitoring room and allows you to talk directly to your father. You tell him you're watching the whole procedure, just to make sure the surgeon does her job right, but if he wants you to, you'll leave for a minute and check on the score of the Cubs game and report back to him. You are both ecstatic and amazed that your father is having the 1995 equivalent of the dreaded coronary bypass while you carry on an everyday conversation as if he were having a wart removed.

The whole procedure has taken only twenty minutes so far, but there is more work to be done. The surgeon removes the holmium laser catheter and immediately inserts another catheter. The nurse tells you that on the tip of this catheter is what is called an ultrasound transducer. By bouncing sound waves off the interior of the coronary artery, the surgeon will be able to see a two-dimensional image of the narrowed portion after the occlusion just opened. First she will measure its extent and then use the ultrasound image—which is also projected onto the monitor for everyone involved to see—as a guide to widening the internal diameter of the coronary artery.

In order to do this, the surgeon removes the ultrasound and introduces yet another catheter. The nurse explains that, because of the extensive calcification detected on the MRI done earlier, the instrument being used here is ideal. You are advised to watch the monitor closely since the results are going to be dramatic.

The catheter is threaded through the new laser-created opening in the blood vessel to where it reaches the beginning of what we can now see is a long and irregular narrow segment of the artery.

On the outside of the catheter is a tiny cylindrical wheel that begins to rotate very rapidly when the surgeon activates a switch. The nurse tells you that this instrument is called a Rotablator and that the whirring component is a wheel covered with more than one thousand tiny diamonds to act as an abrasive. Rotating at more than fifty miles per hour, it is the best of several new instruments called atherectomy devices, designed to mechanically remove calcified plaque from the walls of arteries.

As the surgeon slowly advances the Rotablator, you can see it literally sanding off the narrow, calcified portion of the artery. Slowly and carefully, she continues along the artery for almost an inch, until normal artery is reached. And just as extraordinary as the way the Rotablator is sanding down the calcified portion of the artery is the way it is preventing all the removed debris from piling up. Like a lawn mower with a bag to catch the grass clippings, the Rotablator has a receptacle in which all the calcified artery fragments are deposited to be disposed of when the Rotablator is removed.

Another look with the angioscope, and the ultrasound shows the image of your father's left coronary artery to be almost perfectly clean!

Now, as the surgeon explains to you and your father, the trick is to keep the artery that way. Having him make the lifestyle changes you've been harping about will no doubt help, but more than that needs to be done. Although the laser and the Rotablator have been used with artistic precision, it is impossible to avoid a little damage to the lining of the blood vessel. This sort of damage is what has been responsible for the 40 percent reocclusion rate following the traditional balloon angioplasty. Damage here has been less, but still enough that, if nothing else were done, some recurrences would be expected.

There is, though, a way to prevent this recurrence. Once again reaching over onto the side table, the surgeon selects another catheter, different appearing from any of the previous ones. It's almost as if she were a golfer, gauging the terrain between the lie of her ball and the green, and then choosing the appropriate club from her bag.

This time, the surgeon is using what is called a stent. As the nurse shows you with a replica, it consists of a balloon catheter onto which has been mounted a meshlike slotted tube. While you watch again on the monitor, the catheter is inserted into the artery that has just been cleaned out with the laser and the Rotablator. When the previously diseased segment is reached, the balloon is inflated. This expands the tube against the inside wall of the artery where it now resembles a workman's scaffolding. The balloon catheter is retracted, leaving only the stent in place.

The surgeon explains that the stent serves more of a purpose than just to keep the artery expanded, although that is a very important part of its function. Since there has been some minimal damage to the vessel lining, it will almost certainly initiate the formation of a blood clot, followed by growth of connective tissue cells and smooth muscle cells from the arterial lining. Without the stent, this process would continue until the artery was closed up again. But the stent can serve as a kind of surrogate artery wall, allowing all the clotting and tissue growth to take place on the surface of its scaffolding, sparing the artery from closing up again.

The nurse tells you that implanting a stent in the artery following laser and atherectomy surgery will reduce the chances of the artery closing up again from the 40 percent seen with the typical balloon angioplasty to 10 percent or less. But there is one more tool in their bag to reduce the chance of this happening to zero.

It's not another catheter device but an additional facet of the stent that was just implanted. Although the clotting will take place primarily on the mesh scaffolding of the stent, studies have shown that sometimes it can also occur on the arterial lining, initiating the reocclusion process the surgeon is trying so hard to avoid. So, impregnated into the stent is a genetically engineered drug that acts as a lubricating oil for the blood vessels. It has two components, both of which will be responsive to the deposition of platelets (the small blood cells that are the first sign of clot formation) on the inner wall of the artery. One component of the drug will adhere to the wall of the artery to keep the platelets from attaching, while the other will stay within the interior of the vessel to keep the platelets from loitering where they aren't wanted. The stent itself is biodegradable, designed to slowly deteriorate over a three-month period—the period when the artery is most vulnerable to closing up again—all the while releasing small, measured doses of the novel anticoagulant.

Your father's right coronary artery is treated in the same way as his left has been, except that since there was no acute closure, the laser isn't needed. With the stent and the anticoagulant in place, your father can look forward to many more years of disease-free happy life. And the use of the stent to act as a drug delivery system is merely a prelude to how catheterlike devices are going to be used by the beginning of the next century.

In 1995, not everyone will be fortunate enough to have an impending heart attack prevented with this new high technology. But, because of this technology, the rate of second heart attacks will drop dramatically.

These minimal intervention techniques will be augmented by several other advances, beginning with better diagnosis. It is well known that the earlier an actual heart attack can be detected, the earlier therapy can be instituted and the less will be the residual damage to the heart muscle normally fed by the blocked artery.

When patients with chest pain appear in the emergency room today, the standard way of determining if they have had a heart attack is to hook them up to an electrocardiogram and look for the characteristic changes that every medical student learns. In addition, serial blood samples are drawn every several hours for a couple of days to measure the level of a heart muscle enzyme that is usually released into the bloodstream during a heart attack. This helps detect attacks that aren't seen on the electrocardiogram and confirms those that are. While these tried-and-true methods have proven dependable, they are not infallible. Furthermore, they give unreliable information as to the extent of the damage, and no information at all about the location of the damage—crucial pieces of data if subsequent therapy is to minimize permanent damage to the heart muscle.

To improve the speed of diagnosis, there will be in standard use by 1993 a simple and cheap kit that will detect in ten minutes whether or not a heart attack has occurred. The kit will consist of latex particles coated with an antibody to myoglobin, a protein that is released into the blood soon after a heart attack, often within one hour. On a glass slide, a technician will mix just a drop of a patient's blood with the coated particles and, after only a ten-minute wait, will have a diagnosis faster than any of the methods being used today can deliver one.

It has been known for some time that myoglobin levels in the blood are elevated early in a heart attack, but the methods for analyzing it are too slow to make them practical for routine use. The introduction of the latex kit will make measuring myoglobin levels in the blood standard, and combined with the electrocardiogram and enzyme test routinely employed, the kit is going to improve the sensitivity of diagnosis of early heart attack.

If a heart attack has occurred, doctors today have several ways of gauging how well the patient's heart is functioning as a whole posttrauma, but there is no reliable method for pinpointing exactly where the damage has occurred and how much there has been. By 1995, there will be two new methods to do exactly that, both of which are more complex than the simple test to diagnose the presence of a heart attack.

The first will use a combination of monoclonal antibodies and an imaging technique called a SPECT scan, a more sophisticated version of a CAT scan, one that can detect metabolic changes in tissue. The monoclonal antibodies will be prepared to target a specific portion of the heart protein myosin and will then be labeled with a safe, fast-deteriorating radioactive compound. These will then be injected into already-diagnosed heart attack patients and they will quickly home in on the damaged heart muscle. Thirty minutes later, the SPECT scan will be done and the radioactivity detected will reflect both the location and the amount of damage.

The second method, yet another application of MRI imaging technology, will be easier to use and will employ no radioactivity. In this case, the radiologist will actually take a movie of the damaged heart. The elegant technique, now being developed at Johns Hopkins University Medical School, will use a special tagging procedure to produce detailed images of the heart muscle as it beats and twists. By comparing it with images of a normal heart at work, we will be able to localize and measure the damage.

The early diagnosis of heart attacks and the more precise location of heart damage means that we will be able to treat the heart attack more effectively. One of the major breakthroughs in cardiovascular disease in the 1980s was the routine use of thrombolytic therapy, the intravenous administration of clot-busting wonder drugs as soon after the diagnosis of a heart attack as possible. By dissolving the clot in the obstructed coronary artery and reestablishing blood flow to the starved muscle as soon as possible, this therapy has markedly reduced the death rate from heart attacks, from 30 percent in the 1960s to 10 percent today. Followed by angioplasty, second heart attacks have become much rarer, too.

Ten percent is still too high a figure, though, equivalent to more than 150,000 deaths annually in the United States alone. In just the next five or six years, we can look forward to a more than 50 percent decline in this death rate. With their new diagnostic knowledge, physicians will be able to administer clot-breaking therapy earlier. This will play a significant role in saving lives. So will the laser and the other new technologies used after the thrombolytic therapy.

But there will also be improvements in the clot-dissolving therapy itself. Some of the achievements will be as a result of better drugs to do the job. Created by biotechnology, these new drugs will sharply focus on more specific components of the clotting and anticlotting chemical cascades. This not only will boost the efficacy of the therapy, but even more important will eliminate postdrug bleeding, a major complication with the drugs in use now.

In addition to the risk of bleeding, there is another grand problem with clot dissolution: the threat of hazardous and ubiquitous chemicals called free radicals. This involves the entire mechanism by which heart attacks are caused and what happens when the blocked coronary arteries are opened up by administering the clot-busting drugs. After the heart attack, dangerous things happen on each side of the dammed-up coronary artery. In the heart muscle, biochemical changes take place that use up the normally present supply of antioxidants. Antioxidants, as we mentioned in connection with cancer, are enzymes and nutrients such as vitamins E and C which protect against free radicals.

The depletion of the antioxidants in the heart muscle is dangerous enough in itself, but it is complicated by what happens on the other side of the blockage. Because of the conducive environment behind the dammed-up blood vessel, free radicals congregate in huge numbers, secretly plotting against the heart. When the clot-dissolving drug is administered, the dam breaks, allowing supposedly nourishing blood to flow once again to the hungry muscle. But this blood brings along with it some very unwelcome visitors: a torrent of free radicals. With their natural antioxidant enemies depleted by the pathology that has already taken place in the muscle, the free radicals are virtually unopposed in their effort to wreak biochemical havoc, causing more damage than the initial heart attack itself. This destruction of tissue, called reperfusion injury, may not manifest itself for several months or even years, but these diabolical molecules definitely weaken the heart for the future.

Scientists have conclusively demonstrated this in the laboratory, and there is a body of strong evidence developing that this same sequence takes place when humans have a heart attack and are subsequently treated with clot-dissolving therapy. Many have predicted that if something isn't done to prevent the onslaught of free radicals, it will ultimately prove to be a case of the cure being worse than the disease. For this reason, by 1995, added to the new and better drugs used to break up clots in the coronary arteries will be powerful, computer-designed, synthetically created novel antioxidants.

As extraordinary as all the benefits are going to be from lasers, genetically engineered clot-dissolving drugs, and artificial hearts which will finally come of age, the real breakthroughs in the prevention and treatment of coronary disease are going to occur at the molecular level. Our bodies are beautifully designed to avoid heart attacks. The fact that our lifestyle indiscretions, and occasionally our genes, override nature does not detract from the beauty of the grand plan.

We've already seen how antioxidants are going to play an important role in preventing free radical damage after a heart attack. But antioxidants will have an additional, preventive role to play: they will be used to actually thwart atherosclerosis.

We've all heard about LDL cholesterol, the so-called bad cholesterol, the material that can be deposited in the lining of our arteries. Most experts believe such deposition to be the first step in the buildup of plaque, the substance that, if enough accumulates, can eventually choke off our coronary arteries and cause a heart attack. As you might expect, though, the story is not that simple, and that's where antioxidants come in.

The LDL, or low-density lipoprotein, is really a large particle that ferries around more than just cholesterol in the bloodstream. It carries other fatty substances such as triglycerides, proteins and, somewhat surprisingly, vitamin E.

What's vitamin E doing there? We are beginning to understand that vitamin E is part of the body's master plan. This is by no means a coincidence of evolution. Recent research has shown that not all LDL particles have the same propensity to deposit their plaque-forming cholesterol in the artery wall. A biochemical alteration is required for deposition to occur. Effecting this alteration is our old nemesis the free radical. Since, as by-products of our own metabolism (as well as cigarette smoke, radiation and a high-fat diet), free radicals are floating around in our tissues all the time, the cholesterol in the LDL particle is in constant peril of being converted into a form that the arterial wall can then beckon as tantalizingly as the Sirens called out to Odysseus.

Enter vitamin E, the knight in shining armor. It is tempting and logical as part of the master plan to assume that vitamin E, a powerful antioxidant, has taken up residence in the LDL particle primarily for the purpose of protecting it from attack by free radicals.

Some recent research bears this out. Sophisticated laboratory investigations using monoclonal antibodies as diagnostic tools have discovered that free-radical-modified cholesterol is indeed an integral part of the plaque that closes off arteries, but cholesterol that hasn't been changed by free radicals isn't. In experimental trials, rabbits given an antioxidant drug didn't develop atherosclerosis while on a high-cholesterol diet, whereas those on the same diet but not given the drug did develop atherosclerosis. And, in humans, careful epidemiological studies have shown that one's blood level of vitamin E is at least as good a predictor of risk of subsequent coronary disease as is the blood level of cholesterol itself. In the case of vitamin E, it is a low blood level that increases risk.

More studies are being conducted to home in on the elaborate molecular mechanism involved in protecting the cholesterol from being modified. When this work is done, we are going to see a slew of new and highly targeted antioxidant drugs on the market specifically designed to biochemically protect us against atherosclerosis.

Certainly cholesterol plays a big part and is an integral component of every plaque that encumbers every narrowed artery, but now scientists are looking as well at the soil in which the cholesterol is deposited—the wall of the artery—rather than the seed itself, the cholesterol.

There is some evidence that atherosclerosis may be caused by a virus, much like colds, measles, AIDS and sometimes even cancer. Experts differ on this, however. Arterial tissue taken from patients with hardening of the arteries is frequently infected with a virus called cytomegalovirus, a member of the herpes virus family. But it still isn't clear whether the virus actually plays a role in causing atherosclerosis or is simply an innocent bystander. Eighty percent of Americans are infected with the ubiquitous virus, so it's quite possible that it's merely along for the ride. On the other hand, in a disease as common as atherosclerosis, it would be expected that most people would carry the agent that caused it.

Another feature of cytomegalovirus that fits with it being a perpetrator of coronary disease is that it can remain dormant in cells for a long period of time. An additional infection, or perhaps damage from cigarette smoke, or high blood pressure, could awaken the virus. The belief among proponents of a viral origin is that, when it does become activated, the cytomegalovirus can damage the endothelial cells, the ones that line the coronary arteries. Like a molecular sandpaper, the viral damage roughens the surface of the cells, making it easier for free-radical-altered cholesterol to be deposited, setting the rest of the plaque-forming process in motion. This helps explain why coronary disease often occurs without high blood levels of cholesterol.

The best way of preventing a viral disease is with a vaccine. But a vaccine based on a weakened strain of the cytomegalovirus won't do much good, since most of us with healthy immune systems already have some level of antibodies against this widespread organism and will need something more potent. The portion of the virus that most effectively stimulates the production of antibodies capable of neutralizing the virus will have to be identified and isolated. Then, using genetic engineering techniques, this fragment will be amplified and made into an inoculable form. The antibodies that result from such an injection will be capable of killing off all or most of the potentially dangerous cytomegalovirus in the cells lining the coronary arteries, thus eliminating a major risk for plaque formation. We will have this vaccine within ten years.

Immune intervention is also going to work against coronary disease in those for whom viruses don't play an important role. So far in this drama we've seen cholesterol acted upon by free radicals. This is villain number one. Then we saw the arterial wall acted upon by a virus to become irresistible to cholesterol deposits. This is villain number two. But in addition to cholesterol and the arterial wall, there is a third important villain in the coronary disease drama: the cells that actually engulf the cholesterol.

These cells, a specialized type of white blood cell called monocytes, act first as merely an intermediary, transporting the activated cholesterol a short distance to the lining of the artery. It turns out, though, that once the baton has been passed to them, these white blood cells produce a whole series of molecules that take atherosclerosis to the next level. Here scientists are finding another opportunity to intervene and interrupt the chain of events.

So eager apparently is the activated cholesterol to be shuttled to the lining of the artery that it initiates its own mode of transportation. The cholesterol stimulates the release of a group of immune proteins called "complement," which in turn summon the white blood cells to the scene. Once they arrive, the white blood cells take on their cholesterol passenger and carry it to the artery lining.

Research in laboratory animals has shown that by administering substances that prevent the release of these immune proteins, the necessary white blood cell carriers can be dissuaded from coming to the area, and so the activated cholesterol is left stranded, with no way to get to the artery lining. The development of atherosclerosis is frustrated.

The antiimmune compounds used up until now have been tried only on experimental animals and are too nonspecific for practical use, but the demonstration of the principle means that, before the end of the decade, we will have specific anticomplement antibodies, directed only at the immune fragments that are activated by free-radical-primed cholesterol. This will complete our arsenal for a multipronged attack on coronary disease.

But as targeted and sophisticated as these approaches are going to be, there will still be instances in which the disease eludes the traps being set for it. There will be times when cholesterol will be activated by free radicals *before* the antioxidants can stop this from happening. Viruses will titillate the artery lining before we can get rid of them with a vaccine. And the white blood cells will brave hell and high water to carry out the first phase of their mission, and will happily bring the activated cholesterol to the artery wall. What then?

We will then have reached a new stage in the battle against molecules. Once the white blood cells have been successful in delivering the cholesterol, they give up their nomadic life and take up residence in the wall of the artery along with their passenger. And in order to make certain they won't be evicted, these white blood cells begin producing a series of molecules that markedly accelerate the atherosclerotic process.

First, they find it so comfortable in the lining of the artery that they want to tell all their friends about it. They accomplish this by inducing the cells that line the artery to produce a molecule called an adhesion factor, which makes it far easier for subsequent cholesterol-laden white blood cells to find their way into what will be their new home. Once there, the new colony of white blood cells generate further molecular mayhem. They now instruct the cells of the artery lining to help produce products with names such as platelet-derived growth factor and fibroblast growth factor. Growth factors stimulate the growth of smooth muscle cells in the artery wall, which cause the plaque to expand in size dramatically and practically close off the artery. As this process continues it is likely to cause a heart attack.

Dr. Elizabeth Nabel, a cardiologist and molecular biologist at the University of Michigan, is developing one of the most innovative and exciting techniques to stunt the growth factors. It involves the sophisticated molecular alteration of the internal milieu of the coronary artery where atherosclerosis develops. Dr. Nabel's research has until now centered on how to prevent the restenosis, or the reclosing, of coronary arteries after angioplasty, but it has implications that are much broader.

Since this research is still in the laboratory stage, we won't be ready to modify growth factors routinely on patients for at least ten years, but the research itself is so tuned in to the molecular basis of coronary disease that it is going to provide one of the most important weapons in its early prevention and treatment. When treatment becomes available, catheters will introduce therapeutic genes which will prevent growth factors from working overtime and closing off the artery. Eventually the same homing techniques being developed for cancer gene therapy will be used. A gene will be injected into the patient by a nurse and, because it will be linked to specific monoclonal antibodies, will be like a bullet delivered to the cells lining the coronary arteries.

There will also be new approaches to the problem of high blood pressure, an important risk factor not just for coronary disease but for stroke. An estimated fifty million Americans have high blood pressure, and while in recent years our knowledge of what causes hypertension and how to treat it has expanded tremendously, we are still in need of future breakthroughs, which we'll see in the next decade.

Drugs such as beta-blockers, effective to a degree but with a host of side effects, including depression, fatigue, impotence in men and elevation of blood cholesterol levels, have been replaced with newer agents called ACE inhibitors. These drugs are much more specific in that they work on distinct components of the high blood pressure cycle. Newer molecular therapies will carry this principle much further. The focus will be the endothelial cells that line that artery, the same ones that are the target of the anticoronary-disease molecular therapies of the future.

These versatile cells regularly produce a substance called endothelium-derived relaxing factor or EDRF, which is responsible for keeping the arteries throughout the body in the proper state of relaxation, tense enough so blood can be pumped through them to the tissues but not so tense that they abnormally constrict. When EDRF is inactivated, hypertension can ensue, with all its consequences.

Guess what can, and does, inactivate EDRF? The answer, once again, is free radicals. So free radicals not only can spur on the coronary artery disease process by preparing cholesterol for deposit in the arteries, but also can be a factor in causing hypertension. One of the newest therapies for hypertension in the next decade is going to consist of antioxidants to protect the EDRF from being inactivated, and an alternative strategy will be to administer synthetic versions of EDRF. In addition, there are a whole host of other molecular receptors and hormonelike factors that either are produced by or act on the cells lining the artery that will be molecularly addressed in the treatment of high blood pressure. We can look forward to much better control.

Finally, the molecular and genetic treatment of high cholesterol levels is also on the near horizon. Current estimates are that about 50 percent of high blood levels of cholesterol are caused by diet, the rest by genetic variation. Therefore, the strong emphasis for the past several years on modifying our diets to keep our cholesterol in check has been well directed. But that was before we understood the roles genetics and molecular biology can play. The way cholesterol is regulated is about to change remarkably.

The possible combinations of enzymes, cell surface receptors, proteins and other important molecules involved in cholesterol production and transport are so staggering it's highly probable that each of us has our own unique way of handling fat. By the end of this decade we are going to have a firm hold on identifying the variants of cholesterol metabolism in every one of us. And within five to ten years after that, between 2005 and 2010, we are going to have a number of dazzling new preventive and therapeutic options. Every component of the cholesterol pathway will be adjustable safely and biochemically. Once this is possible, we can, if we wish, revert to our old, and sometimes delightful, bad eating habits. The most wicked among us will no longer be in danger. For those who long for the good old days, molecular biology will be a perfect remedy.

# 8

# Solving the Mystery of Alzheimer's Disease and Other Neurological Problems

BEFORE 1970, ALZHEIMER'S DISEASE WAS AN OBSCURE CONDITION that few Americans lived long enough to encounter. But with the revolution in life extension, this nightmare of old age became a dread force affecting four million people in the United States alone. It has been projected that by 2040, this number will swell to a staggering fourteen million. But it is also clear that over the next twenty-five years, we are going to chip away systematically at the biochemical processes by which Alzheimer's disease is caused until we can treat it and eventually completely prevent it from happening. What's even better news is that in the next four or five years we can expect some early diagnostic tests and before the end of the decade the introduction of drugs that will actually slow down the course of the disease once it is detected. Before 2010 there will be compounds not only to grind the progression of Alzheimer's disease to a halt but to actually reverse it, and by 2020 we will have the molecular means to stop it before it starts. Future scientific histories will describe Alzheimer's disease as a medical problem that existed briefly from 1970 to 2020.

In 1977, in Britain, a series of studies demonstrated that the brain cell death in Alzheimer's disease was not random, as it often appeared to be under the microscope, but rather centered on the cells of what is known as the cholinergic system. The main product of the cholinergic system is the neurochemical messenger (neurotransmitter) acetylcholine, which plays a major role in learning and memory, two functions that characteristically deteriorate in Alzheimer's disease. Since Alzheimer's patients lose much of this important brain chemical, the challenge to research was on to find a means of preserving and supplementing what acetylcholine remained.

Approximately forty separate studies attempted to do this, either by providing natural substances such as choline and lecithin as dietary precursors of acetylcholine or by using drugs to inhibit the enzyme that breaks down acetylcholine. This latter method has been the only one to have any success. An enzyme-inhibiting drug called tacrine or THA (tetrahydroaminoacridine) produced mild improvement in memory and ameliorated confusion. But tacrine, which is marketed under the name Cognex, is not a great drug. Because it is toxic to the liver, the dose can't be pushed high enough to effect any dramatic relief of symptoms.

Queuing up close behind Cognex in the pharmaceutical pipeline are a number of other one-and-a-half generation compounds that do the same thing—inhibit the enzyme that breaks down acetylcholine—but do it more effectively and with fewer side effects. These drugs—Mentane and Synapton are two of them—are the first to provide dramatic relief from symptoms.

Other compounds under investigation take a slightly different approach to the same end—boosting the level of acetylcholine. Some, instead of inhibiting the enzyme that breaks it down, attempt to stimulate the remaining acetylcholine-producing brain cells to work overtime and manufacture more of the chemical. Still others, called agonists, slip into the receptors on the surface of memory and learning cells and trick them into believing the compound is acetylcholine. Both of these approaches are promising, and only about five years away.

How much can we expect from these drugs? It is likely that 40 to 50 percent of patients will experience a significant improvement, pushing back their disease to a level at which they can function partially. This does not, of course, provide a cure, or anything close to one. It doesn't even mean that the course of the disease is slowed. Alzheimer's continues to progress inexorably, but as though it were moved back to an earlier level where fewer dead neurons litter the brain.

What about the 50 to 60 percent of patients who don't respond to these drugs? It is now known that Alzheimer's disease is more than just a deficit of brain cells that produce acetylcholine. A loss of other neurotransmitter chemicals that play a role in memory, learning and cognition (compounds such as norepinephrine and serotonin) is of equal significance.

Therefore, the second generation of Alzheimer's drugs, introduced by 1995, will focus on boosting levels of more than one neurotransmitter chemical. Some of the new drugs will combine, in the same molecule, the ability to augment acetylcholine as well as norepinephrine and serotonin. But there will also be drugs for the augmentation of one compound at a time.

By 1997, fully 80 percent of Alzheimer's patients will experience some functional improvement. This will still be symptomatic improvement only and not a cure. But the progression of the disease will be rolled back further than ever before, giving patients added months and even years of functional life.

It is 1996 and two years earlier, JoAnn and Mike had made the first of their painful decisions and arranged to institutionalize their father in a nursing home. Watching the attendants get him settled in the stark room, their father passively, almost lifelessly complying, they felt the weight of almost unbearable sadness and guilt. But they knew there had been no other choice. For two years after their father had been diagnosed with Alzheimer's in 1992, they had alternated taking care of him in their homes. And it had worked out fine for a while. Dad had had many good days, when he was his old lucid self, displaying his wry sense of humor and the sharp, clever mind that had made him a successful businessman and nationally ranked bridge player.

Those days, though, became rarer and rarer until they finally evaporated completely. For the three months before taking him to the nursing home, their father had spent entire days sitting in a chair, staring at the wall. If Mike or JoAnn or any of their children came into the room, he would look right through them without any display of recognition. He hardly spoke, and when he did it was mostly unintelligible. Finally he reached the point where he could no longer dress himself, feed himself, or even perform his own toilet. They knew what they had to do.

JoAnn and Mike dutifully visited their father twice a week, more to assuage their own consciences than to bring him any cheer. The rides home from the nursing home became increasingly depressing. Having to see this proud and graceful man whom they dearly loved and respected so totally robbed of his humanness was more than they could stand. With each week, what had begun as passing remarks about euthanasia evolved into serious discussion. JoAnn and Mike could hardly believe what they were hearing themselves saying, that they were actually talking about ending their father's life. They had been so close to him all their lives it was almost as if they were contemplating suicide. But they knew they weren't considering it to relieve themselves of the burden. They were absolutely certain their father wouldn't want to exist this way. He had once belonged to the Hemlock Society, the original right-to-die advocacy group, and it had been only with great difficulty that they had convinced him not to end his life when he was first diagnosed with Alzheimer's. Ironically, they were now admitting that perhaps he had been right. They decided to make an appointment with Dad's doctor.

"I certainly commiserate with you, but I don't think euthanasia is the answer right now, and not because it's not legal," Dr. Miller told Mike and JoAnn as they sat in his office two weeks later. "I've just gotten word, kind of insider information if you will, that the FDA is about to approve two new drugs for the symptomatic treatment of Alzheimer's. Remember, these were the ones I told you about last year? We didn't think the approval would come this quickly, but there's been a lot of pressure from activist groups, thank God. And the FDA commissioner is really the best we've ever had. Compared with the old ones, he moves with the speed of light."

"Is it possible these drugs could really help Dad?" Mike asked skeptically. "And even if they could, how much? I don't know when's the last time you've seen Dad, but he's become a vegetable. It's really worse than his being dead. It's hard for me to believe that at this stage anything could help him.'"

Dr. Miller paused and stared down at the desk. "I've been your father's doctor, friend and even occasional bridge partner for fifteen years," he said quietly. "It absolutely devastes me to see him this way, but I look in on him a few times every week. I agree with you he's pretty far gone, but there were patients in the last two studies with these new drugs who were in a similar state and who responded quite well. So I think there's room for some guarded optimism.

"On the other hand, I don't want to get your hopes up too high. There has been some exciting research in the past several years, but even though I'm sure the drugs are going to be approved within a few months, they're still kind of experimental. Without some sort of track record, we just can't accurately predict how or even if he'll respond. But really, what have we got to lose?

"I'll tell you what. Although I've never supervised a euthanasia and I'm pretty uncomfortable with the whole idea, especially in this case, I promise you that if we don't see a response within three months after beginning the drugs, I'll put you in touch with someone."

When Mike and JoAnn agreed with the plan, Dr. Miller told them something else. "One more thing. I want you to clearly understand that this is not a cure for Alzheimer's disease. If these drugs work well, you're going to see a remarkable improvement in your dad's condition. Do you remember the way he was about three years ago? That's the best we can hope for."

"Three years ago!" JoAnn practically shouted with joy. "Dad was living with me then and doing wonderfully. About five days out of every week we watched TV together, argued about politics and even played some two-handed bridge. If he could be brought back to that condition, it would be nothing short of a miracle."

"I agree with you," answered Dr. Miller. "It would be a spectacular turnabout. But do you place a time limit on miracles?"

When Mike and JoAnn looked perplexed, the doctor explained that since this was not a cure, the destruction of brain cells would continue and eventually their father would end up again the way he was today.

"How long?" asked Mike.

"Of course, I can't be certain, but my guess would be that you'd have him back for about two years, three tops. Then he'll begin to deteriorate just as he did a few years ago. You'd have to go through the pain all over again. Maybe it would be too tough on you."

"It's not our pain we're concerned with here," said Mike. "There's no decision to make. We'd go through anything to have our father back for another year or two, to give him back his mind. Start the drugs as soon as you can."

Three months later, the nurses began giving JoAnn and Mike's father two pills every eight hours. Tests had shown that he had deficiencies in two different brain neurotransmitters, and so he was being given a combination drug. Dr. Miller had told them that the average time for seeing any response in the studies conducted was thirty days. Beginning after the first week, either Mike or JoAnn went to the hospital every day and talked to the doctor every other day. After the second week, they both went every day.

On the twenty-second day after beginning the drug, with Mike and JoAnn keeping their bedside vigil, their father recognized them and called them by name. They were without doubt the sweetest words they'd ever heard. Dad still was quite confused and probably didn't understand why they were sobbing and hugging him so tightly.

Over the next two months, he continued to improve and, just as Dr. Miller had hoped, really did come back mentally to where he had been in 1993. During his most rational moments, JoAnn and Mike explained to their father that his recovery was temporary, that someday he would deteriorate again and would probably need to go back to the nursing home. In a conference among all of them, euthanasia was brought up again, since it was on the verge of being legalized. But this time Dr. Miller strongly advised against considering it. As JoAnn and Mike's father's phenomenal rally had demonstrated, researchers were beginning to believe that anything was possible. Even if he did have to be institutionalized again, with proper supportive care it was quite possible that within just a few years there might be new treatments available that could reverse the Alzheimer's for good.

Once again, it was difficult convincing their father. Finally, though, after reminding him that had they not talked him out of suicide five years ago, or had Dr. Miller not convinced them last year that there was something far better than euthanasia, they wouldn't be having this discussion, he acquiesced.

JoAnn and Mike, and their father, treasured every moment of the thirty-one months and twelve days that had been given back. Although they once again had to endure the anguish of seeing him deteriorate, while they could still talk with him they reminded him that it was only temporary, that they had already witnessed one miracle and that even better things were to come.

A far better solution than using drugs to replace lost neurotransmitters would be replacing the actual cells that produce the chemical messengers. This could be accomplished by a brain transplant, a limited implantation of cells carefully prepared in a neuroscience laboratory. The procedure is called neural grafting.

Brain cells grown in cultures and genetically engineered to produce acetylcholine and other neurotransmitters would be surgically grafted into specific regions of the brains of Alzheimer's patients. These cells would not be attached to other cells in the brain. Rather, they would reside in the brain as a sophisticated pharmacological pump that puts out neurotransmitters and never runs dry. Patients no longer would have to take drugs. Once the chemicals were released, their internal homing devices would tell them exactly where to go, even though the implanted cells would exist as an island in the brain tissue. As technically difficult as this may sound, availability of these grafts is not that far away as a treatment. We will see them used within five years.

By 2005, we will have a treatment that will actually send the disease spinning in reverse. We will be able to restore the brain structure to the previous level and even regenerate lost brain cells through the use of proteins called brain growth factors, produced in the laboratory and found to be necessary for neurons to prosper, like food for the brain.

Although the injudicious use of brain growth factors could potentially result in other neural connections going haywire, when these bucking broncos of the brain are properly tamed, they are going to produce some stunning results. But as Dr. Kenneth Davis, chairman of the department of psychiatry at Mt. Sinai School of Medicine in New York, told me, there is no easy way to deliver these to the brain. All of the experiments on Alzheimer's patients have depended on shunts into the brain which remain in place indefinitely, since regularly delivered doses are necessary. So the answer to this problem, Dr. Davis told me, is likely to be the development of *nonprotein* growth factors, compounds that can be taken by mouth, can be absorbed without being destroyed by the digestive juices, and can then cross directly from the bloodstream into the brain.

Because there are many obstacles to be overcome in developing these products, we won't see them used for ten years. But it will be worth the wait. The progress of Alzheimer's disease won't just be temporarily slowed, as with the symptomatic drugs, but will actually be halted and reversed.

• • •

Since it is axiomatic in medicine that the earlier a disease is diagnosed, the greater the chances are for successful treatment, research on diagnosis must keep pace with research on treatment. Every disease that results in organ failure, such as liver or kidney damage, is documented by blood tests that indicate the condition well in advance of the failure. Presently, however, there is no such test for Alzheimer's disease. The only things physicians have to go by are clinical symptoms and a high index of suspicion. As a result, we face inaccurate diagnoses, on the one hand, and late diagnoses, on the other. A diagnosis is frequently made only after Alzheimer's is well advanced.

Fortunately, diagnostic tests for Alzheimer's are on the immediate horizon. Soon we well be able to detect the presence of Alzheimer's in its earliest possible stages. We already know that brain cells begin dying from twenty to thirty years before frank dementia begins—a slow progress. Within five years we will have tests to detect abnormal brain activity that is years away from causing any symptoms of Alzheimer's. This will coincide well with the availability of new treatment. As part of an annual checkup, everyone past the age of fifty will be tested. People with special predisposing circumstances (which we will mention shortly) will be tested at a younger age.

One test may be based on the occurrence of a specific Alzheimer's disease-associated protein in the brain. Dr. Peter Davies, of Albert Einstein Medical College in New York, has developed an antibody to the protein that will detect it in spinal fluid. It will be ready for clinical use within five to seven years. Eventually it will be possible to perform the same test on a blood sample, making it much more comfortable.

New imaging techniques, called PET (positron emission tomography) or SPECT (single photon emission computerized tomography), will also aid in early diagnosis of Alzheimer's. Like the now familiar MRI and CAT scans, PET and SPECT are noninvasive, but they give information about tissue function rather than anatomy. Within seven years, physicians will be able to use them to highlight metabolic changes in the brains of Alzheimer's disease-predisposed patients long before appearance of symptoms.

In 2002, six years after Mike and JoAnn's father was temporarily brought back from the land of dementia, a woman with practically identical symptoms is treated with neurotransmitter replacement.

The therapy is given first by mouth and then, when the desired effect isn't achieved, by a neural graft linked to a circadian computer which delivers a more consistent dose of the chemicals.

This works even better than for the patient in 1996, with remarkable functional improvement lasting almost four years. By 2006, the apparently inevitable deterioration returns. This time, though, the children of this patient do not have to face even the temporary pain of having to return their mother to a nursing home. Six months earlier, oral supplements of brain growth factors had been approved for patient use. Studies had demonstrated that the growth factors could halt, and even reverse, some of the neuron destruction.

With diagnostic tests highly sophisticated by 2006, it is known exactly which growth factors this woman needs to rejuvenate her brain. Within six months after beginning the drugs, her deterioration is arrested, and this time she is here to stay. PET and SPECT imaging scans of her brain, as well as a regularly administered battery of psychometric tests, confirmed the incredible—that indeed she is regaining lost brain cells. She continues to take the growth factor pills for the next twelve years and dies peacefully and independently at the age of ninety-four.

It is a testament to the ingenuity and adaptability of Alzheimer's researchers that they are making such exciting progress in treating the disease without addressing the cause at all. But even the sophisticated, genetically engineered brain cell implants are only high-tech repair jobs. Until the cause is known and addressed, we won't be able to talk of a cure or prevention.

We are getting very close to that time. Using the high-tech molecular methodologies available today, neuroscientists are now learning how to look right inside the brain cells of an Alzheimer's patient and discover what happens at the biochemical level. It's going to be the clinical application of this knowledge that will finally allow us to prevent Alzheimer's from ever occurring.

Ever since German neurologist Alois Alzheimer described the first case in the early 1900s, it's been known that a protein called beta-amyloid is part of the pathology of Alzheimer's disease. Looking at a microscopic section of the brain of a patient who died of Alzheimer's reveals plaques of the homogeneous pink-staining amyloid peppered diffusely over the entire slide. What hasn't been known until recently, though, is whether the amyloid is there as part of the cause of Alzheimer's or just an innocent bystander. Now we know it's a perpetrator.

We're a few years yet from knowing all the precise details, but here's how the Alzheimer's scenario is shaping up. Under normal circumstances, we all produce amyloid, not just in our brain, but in several other tissues as well, where it is important in cell growth. In those unfortunate people destined to develop Alzheimer's, though, the production of amyloid goes slightly astray. The best bet is that an abnormal brain enzyme is responsible for the abnormal amyloid. The derangement in the important enzyme is likely to be just a tiny molecular deviation, such as one amino acid building block exchanged for another. Nature is replete with examples of how unforgiving it is for small errors, and the enzyme missing the mark by just one molecule could have a devastating effect on a life.

Once produced, the abnormal amyloid wanders onerously about in the brain, a toxic shard looking for a way to cause damage. It finally meets a willing coconspirator in the form of a neurotransmitter called glutamate. This chemical is present in all brain cells and, when kept in balance, helps keep all our mental processes running smoothly. The amyloid, though, seduces this neurotransmitter into overstimulation and it quickly undergoes a Dr. Jekyll to Mr. Hyde transformation. By unleashing a series of biochemical reactions in the brain cells it is attached to (mediated once again by the dangerous free radicals), it throws the metabolism of the neuron into irreversible disarray, culminating in cell death. The agonal dance of the brain cells releases more glutamate, additional targets for the diabolic amyloid. And so a chain reaction of neuronal death ensues. This is Alzheimer's at the molecular level.

At the root of all the molecular destruction is likely to be a gene, or more likely a set of genes. That a gene could predispose to Alzheimer's was first discovered in patients with Down's syndrome. With medical advances, many sufferers of Down's syndrome who would have died in their teens and early twenties now live into their forties and fifties. A high percentage of them develop Alzheimer's disease, and the gene responsible was recently identified.

There are also people without Down's syndrome who develop Alzheimer's at this relatively young age, and reseach has now shown that they carry the same gene. Since most cases of Alzheimer's develop much later, it's virtually certain that there is at least one more predisposing gene. Very likely it will turn out to be as many as five or six separate genes that play a part in the production of the abnormal enzyme in the brain that, in turn, produces the abnormal amyloid protein, setting the deadly molecular cascade in motion. Given the breakneck speed at which scientists are working these days, this sequence is going to be known very shortly. What we are working our way toward is a whole series of new compounds to intervene at various points in the molecular pathway that leads to Alzheimer's.

It is early spring 2017 and Andre is having his annual physical. He has been in excellent health for all his forty-four years, but when he was thirty-five a new blood test was introduced to detect the presence of genes that predispose to Alzheimer's. Andre's physician recommended that all his patients take the test, especially those who had a family history of the disease, which was Andre's situation.

Andre's test came up positive. But Andre's doctor told him that the presence of the gene itself meant only that they would have to be extra-diligent in monitoring him. The following week, he had a SPECT scan and a blood test to look for Alzheimer's-related protein, two early tests to determine whether any brain cell destruction had begun. If it had, Andre would have begun taking brain growth factors immediately. Fortunately, his nervous system anatomy and function were perfect.

Each spring for the nine years prior to 2017, Andre's physician performed the same two tests, always with normal results. This year, though, he told Andre he wanted to add another test to the diagnostic battery. Recently a new kit had been introduced to detect the presence of the abnormal brain enzyme produced by the Alzheimer's genes he carried. If this result were positive, it would provide evidence of an abnormality still at the molecular level, one that could be stopped in its track.

As it turned out, the test revealed that, yes, Andre's Alzheimer's genes were already set in motion. Andre was frightened, but not the way people used to be frightened about Alzheimer's, since effective treatments were already available.

"Don't worry," his doctor told him. "I can practically guarantee that you'll never experience any symptoms. If I were to give you some pills, and tell you they were for something else, you'd never even know that your Alzheimer's genes were activated."

Then the doctor explains that he is going to take a multitiered approach, based on the knowledge of exactly what happens in the brain cells to kill them. "First off," he explains, "we're going to try to block the effects of your abnormal enzyme. The enzyme is called clipsin, so the drug has been named clipsin-inhibiting factor. It's a highly specific, computer-designed molecular compound, which will go right to your brain when you swallow it and stop the clipsin. If it works perfectly, no abnormal amyloid protein will get made, and no biochemical mayhem will occur in your brain cells.

"But just in case it doesn't work perfectly, there are two other drugs I want you to take, substances that work slightly further down the molecular cascade. One is called a glutamate antagonist, something we've found useful in a number of neurological diseases. It fits into the receptors on the surface of the brain cells and blocks the effects of the chemical messenger glutamate. If we weren't able to effectively block your brain enzyme, and enough amyloid did get produced, it could conceivably overstimulate this neurochemical which could ultimately kill brain cells. This glutamate antagonist will be another way we can break the cycle.

"Finally, we're going to add a drug called idebenone. Idebenone is an antioxidant and will serve as our final defense, kind of like the free safety on a football team. If the dangerous compounds are somehow able to snake their way through the defenses we've set up, they will try to produce free radicals, which is the last blow before the cell dies. Idebenone will stop this from happening.

"So, you see, we have several ways of ensuring that nothing bad happens to you. We will, of course, continue to monitor all your brain functions, including the activity of your brain enzymes. It will provide us with a barometer of how well our strategy is working. And as effective as this is going to be, it's not even the last word. Five years from now, if you need it, we will be able to give you genetic therapy. In the areas of your brain most sensitive to Alzheimer's we'll be able to implant cells with the gene to produce a normal brain enzyme. This would eliminate all possibilities of Alzheimer's for good."

——— PROGRESS AGAINST PARKINSON'S DISEASE ———

Whereas the neurotransmitter deficits in Alzheimer's disease have been known only since the late 1970s, we've known since the early 1960s that Parkinson's disease is due to a deficiency in the brain neurochemical messenger dopamine. This discovery changed everything. By the late 1960s, high doses of a drug called L-dopa were able to boost levels of dopamine and markedly reduce symptoms of Parkinson's. No matter what their degree of disability, patients responded. Those who had previously been chair-bound or bed-bound by their disease became mobile with the drug. Parkinson's disease became the first neurodegenerative disease to be treated effectively by neurotransmitter replacement therapy and in fact has served in many ways as a prototype for Alzheimer's treatment.

The use of L-dopa was similar to what we are soon to see in Alzheimer's disease, palliative treatment which relieves symptoms but doesn't address the underlying cause of the condition. But L-dopa worked so well for Parkinson's compared with previous treatment, there seemed little interest in further study of the mechanism by which the disease was caused and in development of more specific and effective treatments. As anyone who has had to witness a loved one's speech and movements deteriorate from Parkinson's can attest, it is a serious, debilitating condition. But with most mental processes remaining intact, as a devastating disease it can't be considered in the same league with Alzheimer's. Most researchers were satisfied that Parkinson's was being handled adequately.

Ironically, it was the drug culture that provided the impetus for further progress. In 1983, many people who used a hallucinogen called MPTP rapidly developed a Parkinsonlike disease with marked depletion of dopamine from their brain. They became a model for studying the disease, and it was found that the pathology in these young drug users was the same as in true Parkinson's disease, which comes on far more gradually and in much older people.

MPTP itself is not a neurotoxin. It must first be converted by an enzyme into an active form, which then kills the dopamine-containing nerve cells. Again demonstrating how so many seemingly unrelated diseases have similar pathologies at the molecular level, the vehicles of destruction are free radicals.

This understanding led to a long clinical trial in the late 1980s with two antioxidants, vitamin E and the drug deprenyl. The jury is still out on whether vitamin E slows Parkinson's disease, but the results with deprenyl were not equivocal at all. So effective was it that the trial had to be stopped. Although not widely publicized at the time, the treatment of Parkinson's disease with deprenyl was the beginning of a revolution in neurodegenerative disease management. It was the first therapy to slow down one of these conditions rather than just treat symptoms. This approach, of course, is now being applied full-force to Alzheimer's disease research, but at present, deprenyl remains the most effective treatment for any neurodegenerative disease.

It isn't a perfect therapy, though, and there are several new antioxidant drugs under development, in various stages of clinical trials, that will advance the treatment of Parkinson's disease even further. We can expect to see these on the market beginning within two years and continuing until the turn of the century. In addition, nerve growth factors will be used to regenerate dopamine-producing neurons in Parkinson's.

For those not caught early enough for drug treatment or who don't respond adequately, neural grafting is proving to be an exciting option. As with other aspects of Parkinson's disease, this treatment is further along than it is for Alzheimer's, and in fact a variant of what's to come has already been attempted clinically.

About five years ago, neurosurgeons in Mexico City reported the improvement of several Parkinson's patients who had received transplants from their adrenal glands to their brains (a portion of the adrenal gland contains cells that can produce dopamine). Other investigators around the world had trouble duplicating these results, and the focus turned to fetal brain cells, which seemed more successful. This, though, became shrouded in ethical controversy, as in almost all cases the source of fetal cells was aborted tissue and, under pressure from antiabortion forces, the U.S. government has banned funding for fetal cell research.

But technology is providing a way out. The same brain cell cultures that are being genetically engineered for Alzheimer's disease are being modified to treat Parkinson's disease. Eventually, we'll be able to splice in the gene for dopamine. Human clinical trials should begin shortly, and by 1997 these designer cells will be routinely implanted into the brains of Parkinson's patients who need them.

Neural grafting will deliver remarkable improvement for many thousands of people with Parkinson's, but in ten or fifteen years the disease will be detected early enough in virtually all cases so this therapy won't be needed. The experience with the street drug mentioned earlier, the hallucinogen MPTP, not only spawned new treatments for Parkinson's, but also rekindled interest in the cause. For a time, the consensus among epidemiologists was that Parkinson's was an inherited disease, but familial studies were inconclusive. The effect of MPTP on the brain directed attention to the possibility of an environmental insult. Perhaps there was some other compound that did the same thing the hallucinogen did, but worked more slowly.

Nothing specific has yet been identified, although many researchers feel one of the so-called slow viruses may be the culprit. The prevailing opinion is that Parkinson's is a result of a complex inherited pattern which predisposes one to inadequately get rid of some toxin. The two factors working in league cause a slow destruction of the dopamine-producing brain cells until the symptoms become manifest. Within the next ten years scientists will not only determine the genetics of Parkinson's but identify the toxin (or perhaps toxins) and how the two collaborate.

After the genes are identified, blood tests will become available to detect a predisposition at birth, before exposure to whatever the environmental toxin turns out to be. Scientists are also working on perfecting a PET scan to detect a characteristic inclusion (called a Lewy body) in the brains of people who eventually develop Parkinson's. At present PET scans are very expensive, because they require the use of a cyclotron, a piece of equipment that goes for about a million dollars. But, with time, most new technologies are refined and made cheaper. Already there are being developed minicyclotrons and cheaper PET cameras, both of which will lower the cost of the test. An early diagnosis will allow physicians to institute therapy at the earliest possible stage, in most cases even before symptoms appear.

## NEW TREATMENTS FOR STROKES

It is 1992. The paramedics responded to the 911 call with their usual alacrity. "My wife's been acting confused for almost an hour, and now she just fell down and can't get up. She can't even talk. Please hurry."

"I'm almost certain she's stroked out," said one of the paramedics over the cellular phone in their well-equipped EMS van as they sped to the home of the caller. They were talking with the physician on duty in the hospital emergency room.

"I agree," she said. "Just stabilize her and get her in here *stat*."

Within ten minutes after receiving the call, the paramedics were in the home of an elderly couple. The woman was lying on the thickly carpeted bedroom floor, not unconscious, but paralyzed on her left side. The left side of her mouth was drooped and her tongue was hanging out. She couldn't speak. Her husband looked terrified.

"Sir," the paramedic said, "I'm not a physician, but I'm reasonably certain your wife has suffered a stroke. We'll get her to the hospital as soon as we can. You're welcome to ride in the van with us."

The other paramedic checked the woman's vital signs. Blood pressure, pulse and respiration were all stable. The bedroom carpet seemed to have protected her, because she had no obvious lacerations from her fall, nor did she appear to have suffered any broken bones. He inserted a central intravenous line into the subclavian vein under her collarbone and connected her to nasal oxygen before she was taken to the van. Fifteen minutes later they reached the hospital.

The emergency room doctor commended the paramedics for their quick and thorough work and, after a routine neurological exam and some perfunctory blood work, admitted the woman to the intensive care unit. She remained in the hospital for two weeks, and was discharged fully conscious. She never regained use of her left side and was confined to a wheelchair for the rest of her life.

With some minor variations, this scenario is repeated more than a thousand times every day in the United States alone. Stroke is the third leading cause of death in Americans and the leading cause of disability. Thirty percent of the 500,000 victims each year die, and another 30 percent are permanently disabled, often severely. Some lose consciousness and never regain it; others are paralyzed, suffer visual and speech disturbances, reduced coordination, or a combination of these effects.

After the wave of brain cell death has subsided and the patient has stabilized, physical therapy can often help return some bodily function, but that's essentially all that can be offered today to stroke victims, and it's a far cry from a cure. Doctors are as helpless today in limiting the damage from strokes as they once were in treating heart attacks.

We are soon to witness a major change in the way strokes are handled. Several new treatments that will be instituted within the next ten years will cut the death rate by more than 75 percent and the incidence of disabilities even more than that. Combined with the effective stroke prevention measures already in place—control of blood pressure, blood sugar and cholesterol levels, smoking cessation and limiting alcohol intake, all of which will be improved—we will be firmly in control.

Let's imagine the same situation as before, but this time in 1998. The paramedics receive the same distress call and hurry to the scene. After confirming their suspicion that the patient has suffered a stroke, and after starting the intraveneous line, the first thing they do is infuse a 10 cc syringe labeled "glutamate antagonist." This simple procedure, the result of years of molecular research, is going to have an amazing effect on this patient's life. She will recover completely.

The glutamate antagonist is the same drug that eventually will be used as molecular prevention of Alzheimer's disease. Although the mechanism of overstimulation of the neurotransmitter glutamate is different in stroke than scientists are finding with Alzheimer's—lack of oxygen to the cells rather than an abnormal amyloid protein—the result is similar: brain cell death. In the case of stroke, because of how it happens, the whole procedure is tremendously accelerated. Millions, even billions of neurons can die within hours. By injecting the glutamate antagonist, the paramedics are able to provide an effective means of breaking the chain reaction of cell death. These antagonists sprint to the glutamate receptors on still-healthy neurons and fit themselves firmly in place. The glutamate released from the few neurons that were destroyed when the first wave of the stroke hit will find no other free targets.

While on the way back to the hospital, the paramedics are on the phone telling the emergency room physician what they have done. Even though they aren't more than ten minutes away, he instructs them to inject syringes containing two different drugs immediately. Each will provide an additional line of defense, since time is of the essence in limiting molecular damage from a stroke.

The first syringe the paramedics reach for contains dextromethorphan, a common ingredient used for decades in cough syrup, which has now found a much more important application. As a stroke progresses, the glutamate molecules that are successful in anchoring themselves to neighboring neurons open channels in the cell membrane, allowing a flood of calcium to rush in, much more than is needed for ordinary electrical activity of the cell. If unchecked, the excess calcium stimulates the formation of free radicals, which kills the cell. The injection of dextromethorphan plugs the calcium channels and prevents them from opening.

Finally, as the ultimate thwarting step, the paramedics inject two syringes of antioxidants to mop up any free radicals that manage to get produced. The ones chosen are novel antioxidants called 21-aminosteriods and lazaroids, which have the special property of being able to cross the "blood-brain barrier" into the spinal fluid that bathes the brain.

When the paramedics arrive at the hospital with their patient, the neurologist on call is waiting and immediately orders a CAT scan of the brain. This is a crucial step to determine what type of stroke the patient has suffered, something that will effect further therapy.

There are several kinds of stroke, but the two most common are hemorrhagic and ischemic. Hemorrhagic stroke is often the result of poorly controlled hypertension, which progressively weakens the blood vessels in the brain and culminates in a bleeding episode. Ischemic stroke is far more common, the result of long-standing atherosclerosis, which causes a clot to block a blood vessel, depriving the brain of oxygen. It is analogous to an obstructed coronary artery leading to a heart attack.

Although both types of stroke result in the same molecular mechanism of brain cell death—and therefore the injections given by paramedics are helpful regardless of the cause—the next step depends on whether the stroke was ischemic or hemorrhagic.

If the stroke was hemorrhagic, no other therapy would be helpful at the moment. If, on the other hand, the stroke was ischemic, there is a great deal the physician in the hospital can do. The CAT scan differentiates this and shows that the patient has suffered an ischemic stroke. A clot is blocking the carotid artery supplying the brain.

The entire imaging procedure takes only fifteen minutes. Again, time is extremely important. When he gets the results, the neurologist immediately injects directly into the intravenous tubing a measured dose of a genetically engineered anticoagulant. These clot-dissolving drugs have proved to be of much benefit in limiting damage from heart attacks. A large study completed in 1994 confirmed that anticoagulants also worked in stroke. And just as is done with heart attacks in 1989, along with the clot dissolution therapy, the physician adds another antioxidant, to prevent the brain from being overwhelmed with free radicals when the clot is dissolved.

In order to limit the damage to the oxygen-deprived brain as much as possible, it is vital that the clot-dissolving drugs be administered as soon as possible. Unfortunately, in 1998, paramedics have no definitive way of determining in the field whether a patient has suffered a hemorrhagic or an ischemic stroke. Administering an anticoagulant to a patient with a hemorrhagic stroke could be fatal, so they have to wait until they arrive at the hospital and the CAT scan can be performed, not the ideal solution, but the only one available in 1998.

Five years later, though, by 2003, imaging technology will have advanced far enough so that portable imagers will be standard equipment on every paramedic van. The image will be electronically conveyed to the hospital and interpreted, all within a matter of a few minutes. For those patients with ischemic stroke, the clot-dissolving therapy will be administered at the scene. This will limit the aftermath of stroke to almost undetectable molecular damage, something from which victims will recover completely.

For those not reached early enough, or who have a severe hemorrhagic stroke and sustain a large chunk of irreversible brain cell death, there will be some fantastic help available. These people literally have a "hole in their head,'" a cavity in their brain left by the dead neurons. This cavity will now be filled by brain cell transplants. These transplants will be more advanced than the neural grafts used for treating Alzheimer's and Parkinson's disease. Instead of being just a pharmaceutical pump to provide a source of a lost neurotransmitter, the cells implanted in the brains of stroke victims will be expected to be fully functioning brain cells, capable of the same kinds of communication with the rest of the brain as their deceased predecessors. Therefore, they not only will have to continue growing as they did in cell cultures in the laboratory, but will need to make anatomical and biochemical connections with neighboring cells.

How can these cells from tissue cultures have the "wisdom" to do that? The reason neurons, which begin life in the brain as embryonic cells, make these connections in the first place is that the targets they are supposed to grow to—the other parts of the brain—secrete various growth factors which "tell" the young cells in which direction to grow and what kinds of connections to make. The same mechanism will work with the implanted cells. Once the rest of the brain recognizes some potentially friendly new neighbors, they will send out the welcoming committee.

The clinical application of this procedure for stroke victims is about ten years away. When it is available, the results will be nothing short of miraculous. We will see comatose or severely disabled patients returning to normal life.

# 9

# The Next Plague

THE OFFICIAL ANTICLIMACTIC ANNOUNCEMENT OF A DEMO-
graphic fact that will be evident in stages at the end of this decade
will be made in the year 2003. An expert panel on infectious diseases assembled by the World Health Organization will address a
press conference in Geneva to proclaim to the world that the AIDS
epidemic has ended.

For the following five years, until the impact of the new treatments are fully felt, there will still be sporadic cases and deaths
around the world. But the introduction of more than ten new
antiretroviral drugs, beginning in 1993, as well as several highly
potent vaccines will have enabled physicians to attack the HIV
virus at each of its now well-known molecular sites. Global dis-
semination of these products through an unprecedented international cooperative effort will have resulted in effective protection
and treatment in the Third World countries of Africa, Asia and
South America, as well as the inner cities of Western society.
Ninety percent of all cases will be curable and the incidence will
have decreased by 85 percent.

Research on AIDS will have contributed much to the conquest

of other diseases. In the ten-year period, the accelerated deciphering of the molecular workings of the immune system generated by scientists working on a cure for AIDS will have led to precise ways of controlling and preventing most previous "incurable" immunological diseases: rheumatoid arthritis, multiple sclerosis, insulin-dependent diabetes, psoriasis and ulcerative colitis among them.

In the year 2003, a forty-nine-year-old surgeon watches the news conference on television in the doctors' lounge at Stanford University Hospital, and thinks about implications of the operation he will perform in just one hour. As chief of transplant surgery at a major medical center, he has had his share of important cases, and he has contributed significantly to the worldwide body of knowledge on transplantation immunology, but he's never had a real first. But this, he knows, is it. He isn't just performing the first liver xenograft—an animal-to-human transplant of a liver—but this is the first transplant of any organ from an animal that isn't planned as a stopgap measure. The Baby Fay transplant of a baboon heart twenty years ago was intended to be temporary. But today's procedure is expected to work indefinitely. The surgeon feels confident. He's done much of the important clinical research on rapamycin and 15-deoxyspergualin, two new antirejection drugs that will allow for successful xenograft transplantation.

There is still such a woeful shortage of single organs for transplant, like hearts and livers, that surgeons everywhere are hoping animal transplantation will solve the worldwide problem. This operation will be a turning point.

Before long the surgeon plunges his hands into latex gloves, and one of the circulating nurses helps him into his gown and mask. He looks around the room to make sure the whole team is present. Three more attending surgeons, two residents, four nurses and two tissue technicians, perfusing the baboon liver in the Plexiglas container with the cold preservation solution. At 0400 the liver had been removed and put immediately into the Biotime solution and the animal humanely sacrificed by the animal transplant team.

Now, at precisely 0700, the surgeon and his team begin the surgery, removing the fourteen-year-old female patient's congenitally diseased and microscopically malformed liver, kept borderline functioning by amazing new drugs, but eventually running out of gas. The baboon liver is transplanted, bile ducts and blood vessels anastomosed, and the patient taken to recovery. The operation comes off without a hitch. The surgeon is so absorbed during the procedure he doesn't look up once. As the last suture is closed, he comes out of his semitrance, glances at the OR clock and makes a mental note: 1156.

The young patient is given antirejection drugs, along with a monoclonal antibody to fine-tune her immune response against the foreign baboon proteins, and these work even better than the doctor or any of the consulting immunologists expected. A press conference is held at which it is announced that xenografts are now a reality. What no one can possibly know is that the stage has been set for the next worldwide plague.

Before we follow this story further to see how a plague comes of these circumstances, let's pick up a parellel thread and go back to September 14, 1990, when, after several years of brilliant research and tireless lobbying of a host of government agencies, National Institutes of Health researchers W. French Anderson and R. Michael Blaese were finally given the go-ahead to begin what was certain to be a new era in medicine: genetic therapy.

Their first patient was a four-year-old girl with a rare enzyme deficiency disease which prevented her immune system from working properly. Without external replacement of this enzyme she would die. The enzyme, known as ADA, could be injected or transplanted in cells, but neither technique worked well, and each had to be repeated too often to make it practical. The NIH researchers came up with the methodology of removing just those of her immune cells that lacked the enzyme, inserting into the DNA of those cells the gene to make the enzyme, and then returning the cells to her body. The now normal cells wouldn't live forever, so the process would have to be repeated, but only every few months. If everything worked well, the little girl, otherwise sentenced to certain death, would be able to live an almost perfectly normal life.

Everything did work beautifully. There were several keys to the methodology, but the most important turned on how the gene was transferred into the immune cells that needed it. After much experimentation with different methods of gene transfer, the consensus developed that the only reliable method was to use a virus as a courier. Certain viruses have the innate ability to wriggle their way into human DNA. Ordinarily (such as with the HIV virus) this was a contemptible trait, since the virus could then commandeer the cell's genes for its own reproductive purposes, but in this case the scientists were harnessing the property for benefit, not harm.

First, in the laboratory, they introduced the desired gene into the virus. Then the crucial step: the reproductive apparatus of the virus was disabled. Then their custom-designed, emasculated viral messenger was incubated with the cells they had removed from the little girl. The virus insinuated its genes—and along with them, the gene for the enzyme the patient was missing—into the immune cells. These were then injected back into the patient. The virus would do the job required of it, and would be unable to reproduce. Therefore, the entire procedure was perfectly safe.

There was some general uneasiness about this among the new breed of medical ethicists, and among some prominent microbiologists as well, but several experiments convinced the regulatory panels the virus could do no harm. The virus chosen in this case was a mouse leukemia virus, disabled, and not even known to cause disease in humans in its most natural state. The few dissenting voices were largely ignored, drowned out by the aura of tremendous confidence and exhilaration over what was happening. The little girl's parents praised the NIH scientists as geniuses and genetic therapy as a bona fide miracle.

And this was just the beginning. Shortly thereafter, Dr. Steven Rosenberg and his colleagues at the National Cancer Institute were given the go-ahead for a different kind of genetic therapy, the insertion of a tumor-killing gene into the white blood cells of terminal cancer patients. Although the purpose here was to genetically enhance rather than replace a genetic deficiency, the vector used was the same mouse leukemia virus. Once again, the results were considered a huge success. These were patients expected to die within months, even weeks. Several of them gained years of productive life.

Things would move quickly during the rest of the decade. Genetic therapy would become the hottest, most exciting field of science, quickly populated by the best minds in science and medicine, all of whom had their pet recalcitrant conditions to which they wished to apply the new treatment. By 1995, several new journals devoted to the subject would be published.

The ethicists who were monitoring the results in order to keep genetic therapy from becoming an unregulated runaway train insisted that the next efforts be devoted to the incurable diseases, especially those genetically well established to have a simple mode of inheritance. These were conditions such as muscular dystrophy, sickle cell anemia, Huntington's disease, hemophilia and cystic fibrosis.

Scientists had no shortage of material to work with. Novel methods of administering genes were devised, such as aerosol delivery of the corrective genes directly into the lungs of cystic fibrosis patients. In other cases, primitive connective tissue cells called fibroblasts were cultured in the laboratory, genetically modified to suit the disease being treated, and then implanted under the skin of the patient. Even if they weren't the same kind of cells that normally carried the gene, they were able to do the job. Fibroblasts carrying the gene for the clotting factor missing in hemophilia (normally made in the liver) were able to produce enough of it in patients to cure them. In all cases, though, there was one constant. No matter what kind of cells or what the method of administration was, a disabled virus was the vector to transport the gene into the desired cells.

By the late 1990s, genetic therapy was used to treat diseases which not only had more complex genetics but had other, more established modes of treatment. And why not? There had been no serious complications from any of the genetic therapy to date, and the Human Genome Project was rapidly deciphering many disease-related genes. Some cases of elevated blood cholesterol were being handled by virus-delivered genes. So were the conditions of patients who had had angioplasty but who were at high risk for recurrent coronary artery obstruction. Here the viral gene was delivered via catheter. Many cases of cancer were handled with genetic therapy, too, not just terminal cases as in the early 1990s, but more routine ones.

Finally, in the early years of the twenty-first century, genetic therapy would be used preventively, to treat people with genetically diagnosed disease predispositions, but no overt sign of disease. Since so many people had these predispositions, virus-delivered genes would be more commonplace.

And now let's return to the first baboon liver transplant in the year 2003, reported at the surgeon's press conference on every major television and radio network and published in every important newspaper and magazine in the world. Calls from patients with terminal heart conditions and from parents of children with congenital organ malfunction inundated the switchboards of every medical center around the world.

Within the first year after the global program was enacted, more than seven thousand xenografts of hearts, livers and lungs were performed, and by the end of the third year, when things were running much more smoothly, the total swelled to a staggering thirty-six thousand.

On the morning of October 12, 2007, a man we'll call Roy phones in sick to work. Ordinarily, an employee taking a sick day would draw no attention, but Roy is no ordinary employee. A senior account executive at a large Chicago advertising agency, he has never missed a day of work in his entire ten years with the company, except for the month two years ago when he had the heart transplant down at Pritzker Hospital. But even there his performance was amazing. Here was a patient who'd had cardiomyopathy from some virus infection five years earlier, and he'd never even missed a day of work for that. And after the transplant, he was supposed to recuperate at least six weeks to get used to his new baboon heart, but he'd insisted he was fine after just thirty days.

This morning, however, he's stayed home complaining to his wife Laura that he has a headache he describes as a real sonofabitch. His temperature is 103 and he vaguely wonders whether these flulike symptoms could have anything to do with his transplant or the drugs he is taking, but he quickly reassures himself that the drugs are supposed to be so specific that all they work on is the part of the immune system that might reject the baboon heart.

Roy doesn't go into work the next day either, or ever again. The following morning his temperature is a little worse. His wife won't even let him get out of bed.

She calls his doctor. An appointment is made for three that afternoon.

A half hour later, when Roy tries to get out of bed to urinate, he walks two steps and falls over. He feels as if he were drunk. Down in the kitchen, Laura, who had called in to work herself because she was beginning to feel a little feverish and thought she too was catching the flu, hears the thud and bounds up the stairs. But she is so dizzy she has to stop halfway up to grab the banister. Reaching the bedroom, she finds Roy desperately trying to pull himself up off the floor.

Watching him makes Laura even dizzier. She holds on to the dresser. "I think I've got the same bug you do, Roy, and I think your macho bravado's a bunch of crap. I don't want to wait five hours for you to be seen, and I want to be seen, too. I'll help you get dressed and I'm going to call a taxi. We're going to the emergency room."

"That's ridiculous," says Roy feebly, still unable to get up off the floor. But Roy is scared and so is Laura. Laura now decides to call 911.

Ninety minutes later both Roy and Laura are taken from the ER to the intensive care unit, where they are admitted.

"You're both pretty sick," the emergency room physician tells them. "We'll have to wait just a few minutes for the results of your spinal tap, but I'm reasonably certain you guys have meningitis, and maybe even a touch of encephalitis, what with all your lack of coordination. We call that cerebellar ataxia.

"Your white blood cell count isn't that high, and your spinal fluid wasn't too cloudy, so my initial thoughts are that it's a viral meningitis-encephalitis. In any case, as sick as you feel, and really are, these diseases are pretty self-limiting. My guess would be you'll be out of ICU in a day, be discharged from the hospital in five and be perfectly fine in less than two weeks.

"It is a little strange, though. If you do in fact have viral encephalitis, these things are usually carried by mosquitoes, not exactly something you see too much in Chicago in October."

The lab results indeed confirm that this is a viral infection, not a bacterial one. Just to be safe, however, intravenous antibiotics are started. The consulting neurologist sees them the next morning and, when he first examines his patients, is furious he hadn't been contacted the day before. Both Roy's and Laura's condition had deteriorated significantly. They are drowsy, barely responsive. Two hours later Roy becomes comatose, and four hours after that Laura follows suit. Within three days they are both dead.

None of the antemortem or postmortem blood work is revealing, other than that they both had had some kind of infection. A routine viral screen for antibodies discloses nothing. Autopsy reveals an acute meningoencephalitis in each of their brains, but nothing else. Roy's baboon heart is unaffected. As is standard in these cases, the pathologist takes tissues from every organ, freezes it at minus 170 degrees centigrade and sends samples to the Centers for Disease Control in Atlanta.

Upon receiving the samples four days later, the chief of virology is a little surprised. This is the second such case he's heard of in a week, a fulminant, deadly viral meningoencephalitis of unknown causation. He files the frozen specimens in labeled tissue drawers. He is mildly curious but is busy on another project and will get to these possibly next week.

By the following week, the virology lab has much more work to do, and their interest has increased. Ten more cases with the same history have been reported, and the tissue specimens have arrived. Four of them involved married couples. The chief of virology begins to wonder: could there be a viral encephalitis that isn't mosquito-borne, as it usually is? He calls in the epidemiological team.

While the epidemiologists investigate the pattern of all the reported cases, the virologist thaws specimens from several areas of the brains of each of the unfortunate victims, and from Roy's baboon heart. He subjects each of them to the polymerase chain reaction to amplify their genetic sequence and runs them in the computer against known viral nucleic acids. After a point, this is an entirely automated procedure, so once the tissue specimens are prepared, he sets the mechanics in motion and goes home.

Examining the printouts the next morning, he is astounded; as a matter of fact, he can scarcely believe what he's reading.

"Jill, Tom, come in here," he calls over the intercom to two of his staff virologists. "I want to make sure I'm not hallucinating."

The three of them hover over the nucleotide sequence and interpretation the computer has printed out. "No exact match with existing data base. Closest is Bunyavirus." The same sequence has been identified in the brain tissue of every one of the cases and in the baboon heart.

"This is incredible," says one of the staff. "Isn't Bunyavirus an arbovirus, carried by mosquitoes, the cause of that outbreak of California encephalitis in Kern County about thirty years ago? What the hell is it doing showing up on this printout, and why the substitution of cytosine for thymine in the gene sequence?"

"I think we've got a Bunyavirus with a point mutation," answers the virologist. He paces back and forth, rubbing his chin. "You know what's happening? Somehow, every one of these people has been infected by a mutated Bunyavirus, one that has suddenly become much more common and much more virulent."

"Somehow the baboon heart must be the reservoir," says Tom Dempsey, the other virologist. "I seem to remember that apes sometimes harbor a form of Bunyavirus that doesn't cause human disease. But it somehow mutated to where it does."

All three suddenly have the same thought. Checking with the epidemiologists confirms it. Four of the ten cases had been part of the xenograft program. Two had received hearts, one a lung and the other a liver. Gene sequences of those transplanted animal tissues revealed the same mutated Bunyavirus.

The epidemiologists also deduced two other pieces of information equally astounding and frightening. The mode of transmission almost certainly was sexual contact. No co-workers of the transplant patients or other close contacts other than sexual ones were infected. But through sexual contact a chain of infection was slowly created and the disease was spreading.

That could mean only one thing: that the virus had been transplanted from animal organs, mutated in the recipients who were on antirejection drugs, become virulent and then capable of being transmitted sexually, and finally broke out into the general population. The epidemioligists' and virologists' worst fears are confirmed several times over during the next two years when seventy-five thousand people around the world die of viral meningoencephalitis.

And soon a second plague, stemming from the thrilling breakthroughs in genetic therapy we described earlier, could be overwhelming the scientific community.

In 2010, the new cases came trickling in, just as they had with the Bunyavirus plague. The virology department at the Centers for Disease Control received specimens and case reports from all over the world every day, many of them unusual illnesses, but almost always isolated incidents.

This time, though, following an epidemic pattern, the trickle quickly became a steady stream, and then suddenly a torrent. At first, since these patients had suffered from confusion followed by coma just as the thousands of others had, it was assumed these were merely more of the same. But it quickly became clear that wasn't so. In these new cases, the symptoms in the central nervous system developed over weeks, not days as with the Bunyavirus. This was a slower, more relentless progression to death rather than a quick fatal strike. In addition, every one of the case reports accompanying the frozen organs described a marked hemolytic anemia with bizarre fragmented red corpuscles on the blood smear, as well as severe kidney failure: the hemolytic-uremic syndrome. Could this still be the same virus that had once again mutated? All those generations of viral reproduction in all those people. It was possible.

It seemed highly unlikely, though. Not only was the disease different, but the method of transmission was, too. These cases could not be traced sexually by the epidemiologists. Casual contact with co-workers and friends seemed to be the mode of transmission, probably through respiratory droplets, a far more frightening prospect. Every cough or sneeze could contain a potentially lethal virus, just like the influenza pandemic of almost one hundred years before in 1918.

After further probing into the histories of hundreds of cases, the epidemiologists finally determine that the likely origin of this new plague is genetic therapy, the technique that had been hailed worldwide as the greatest advance in medicine in the past one hundred years.

Once again a virus is the vehicle of destruction, but arising in a different manner from the Bunyavirus epidemic. Experts had been correct in predicting that the viruses used as vectors to deliver the genes into the cells that needed them were incapable of reproducing. But what they underestimated was the ability of these apparently harmless viruses to recombine with other apparently harmless viruses already resident in the tissues of the gene recipients. Molecular analysis of the organs from dead patients demonstrates a mutated virus, this time a reovirus often present in human tissues which rarely causes any disease, and certainly never anything serious. Just a slight change in the genetic structure of the reovirus, brought about by combining with the new gene vector, was enough not only to make it capable of causing a deadly disease but to give it a deadly mode of transmission, creating an epidemic.

The scientific community, while trying to reassure the public, is privately in a panic. How could we in 2010, into the greatest era science and medicine have ever known, be struck with not one viral plague but two? Looking back, underneath all the hoopla surrounding tissue transplantation and genetic therapy—all of it deserved—the answers were to be found.

In the early nineties, when this was all getting started, Dr. Edwin Kilbourne, the chairman of the department of microbiology at Mt. Sinai Hospital in New York, as well as other prominent microbiologists, warned us of this. The manipulation of nature always carries some risk, and when we begin to share organs and genes with each other and among different species, we are running a huge potential risk. The immunological and molecular compatibilities may just not be there, as scientists around the world would one day find out and have to deal with.

This was not to say, nor did Dr. Kilbourne suggest twenty years earlier, that the engines of scientific progress should have been shut down. The transplant surgeons and the proponents of genetic therapy had been right. The amount of disease, suffering and death relieved and prevented had been immeasurable.

But you are not in the future as you read these pages. You are in the present, before this miraculous and dangerous journey has begun. Should you try to stop its progress? Not at all. Whatever progress we make in the future will bring with it a price to be paid. This is what happens when nature is challenged. But paying the price will be temporary. When the new plagues come, we will conquer them; be assured.

# 10

# The Future of Everyday Complaints

—————— SLOWING THE AGING PROCESS ——————

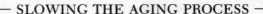

Aging hardly qualifies as a minor annoyance, but since it's something we think about often and from which none of us can escape, it belongs at the head of our agenda. The disappointing news is we're not going to become human sea anemones and live forever. Death will still be the necessary end Caesar predicted. But we are going to be able to postpone the inevitable much longer than most of us would have ever thought possible. And we're going to do it by taking safe drugs every day, beginning when we're still young and healthy.

After years of deliberation, scientists finally agree that aging is a process itself, independent of the diseases that occur as we get older. Even if we never developed cancer, cardiovascular disease, Alzheimer's disease or some other condition associated with senescence, we'd still have to age and die.

Aging is written into our species script; how long we can potentially live is called our maximum life-span, which is currently considered to be about one hundred and twenty years. Since average life expectancy at birth is not even eighty years, this leaves a lot of years to add to our expectations. Given all the advances we're going to see in controlling and alleviating the diseases of aging, achieving theoretical maximum is beginning to be a realistic hope. And once we achieve it, we'll push it further—to one hundred fifty and beyond.

Aging research is still in its infancy, but what's already certain is that one of the causes of aging that we *will* be able to do something about is in our genes. The mechanism we have to combat works in a way exactly opposite to what happens in cancer, where oncogenes, or growth accelerators, are turned up too high and the tumor suppressor genes, which normally act as brakes, are lost. Some very provocative research has found that certain cells age when suppressor genes that control growth are pushed to work too aggressively. The net result is that growth eventually stops altogether, and the cell dies. Eventually it will be possible with targeted drugs to keep our cells alive longer.

Another actively researched approach to maximal longevity is the manipulation of our hormones. We will either have an injection or take a pill of custom-designed hormones that will be able to slow cell metabolism just enough to retard aging without adversely affecting any other functions in our body.

There are also other factors associated with aging, and while we will tame them somewhat, we won't be able to stop them completely. One of them is free-radical damage. Despite our built-in antioxidant protection, injury from free radicals accumulates as we age, and eventually kills our cells. By taking some novel antioxidant protectors, called PQQ and BH4, the ineluctable cell death will be significantly retarded.

Another unavoidable factor is the continual attachment of ubiquitous sugar molecules to proteins throughout our bodies, a chemical process that slows metabolic function and ultimately destroys the cells. This will be impeded with a drug called aminoguanidine.

Although we'll witness an extension of our life expectancy over the next twenty years—to ninety or above—it won't be until at least 2015 that the antiaging research going on today begins to bear fruit. But when it does, there will be a steady increase of our maximum life-span. By 2030, we will be making a media star of the first human to have lived to one hundred fifty. And it won't stop there.

—————— MOLECULAR BIOLOGY TO CURE ALLERGIES ——————

Except for anaphylaxis—that immediate, life-threatening and fortunately uncommon reaction to insect stings and certain foods—most allergic reactions are only nuisances. But to those who have to endure a constant runny nose, itchy eyes and sneezing with every change of season, pollen and grasses, or every time they come near a dog or cat, the nuisance is a major one that affects both productivity and pleasure.

If you're one of those who suffer from allergies, you also know that, despite the best efforts of the medical profession, the treatment and prevention of environmenal allergies have fallen short of being effective. You submit to extensive, and expensive, allergy shots and take antihistamines and other drugs. They sometimes help, but rarely enough.

Using many of the same techniques of molecular biology that are being employed for several of the more serious diseases, allergists and immunologists are predicting considerable breakthroughs in therapy for allergic reactions, both minor and severe.

Allergies result when an offending substance called an allergen (a protein from a plant, animal or food) enters the body. There it hooks up with a special kind of antibody called IgE. This combination now attaches to receptors on the surface of equally distinctive white blood cells. The result is a string of reactions that lead to the familiar annoying symptoms.

Immunologists have already developed a monoclonal antibody to attach to the IgE floating around in our bloodstream. When injected either regularly for a chronic allergy, or when needed to prevent a severe, acute reaction such as to a bee sting, the antibody binds to the IgE and will prevent the IgE from binding with an irritating allergen should we come in contact with it, and there will be no symptoms. Although we need some IgE (primarily to fight parasitic infections), allergic people have an excess of IgE, much more than they need for normal health. And binding up the IgE won't prevent our other antibodies from being available to protect us. Animal trials with this monoclonal antibody have been encouraging, and human trials are about to start. We can expect to enjoy the full benefit of this treatment by 1998.

A variation on this same theme is the development of drugs or other monoclonal antibodies to block the receptors on the surface of the white blood cells involved in allergic reactions. Even if all the IgE molecules available aren't handcuffed and some manage to combine with the allergy-producing substances after they enter our body, blocking the receptors will keep them from setting off the damaging cascade.

This type of immunotherapy is different from what allergists use today in that it is nonspecific, that is, the monoclonal antibodies or the drugs will tie up whatever free IgE we have floating around, or whatever receptors are on the cells, regardless of what it is we're allergic to. But there will also be marked improvements in the specific end of the allergy equation, desensitizing us to particular substances.

One of the reasons allergy shots have not been more effective is that the material prepared for injection hasn't been pure enough. Molecular biologists and chemists are coming up with ways to refine the preparation process to produce exactly the material they want— cat allergen, ragweed, or whatever else we're sensitive to. Then, by conjugating these pure proteins with polymers such as poly-ethylene glycol and injecting them, allergists are learning how to block the production of any IgE antibodies against these proteins. Combining these two types of treatment will mean highly effective relief for almost all of us with allergies.

## DRUGS TO STOP MIGRAINES
### —————— ALMOST IMMEDIATELY ——————

Fifteen years ago, while spending a night in a Holiday Inn in Columbia, South Carolina, I was jolted out of a sound sleep with the only migraine I've ever had, a throbbing pain and nausea so intense I'll never forget it. I went to a local emergency room and had a shot of Demerol, which helped, but not quickly enough. It took about six hours, which seemed like sixty, before I was rid of the migraine.

If this has ever happened to you, or if you're more unfortunate and are among the millions who suffer regularly from migraines (eight million in the United States alone), I'm sure you can visu-alize, even feel, exactly what I mean. Your troubles, though, are about to end.

Several studies reported in 1991 that injections of a drug called sumatriptan were remarkably effective in alleviating pain, nausea and vomiting from migraines within less than one hour after administration. It worked beautifully in 75 percent of the hundreds of people in the clinical trials.

Sumatriptan is a compound that activates chemicals that increase the effect of the brain neurotransmitter serotonin. The role of serotonin in migraines isn't perfectly understood yet, but somehow those predisposed to migraines have low levels of serotonin in their blood. These reduced levels trigger a dilation of blood vessels to the brain, accounting for the characteristic throbbing and other symptoms. By increasing the amount and effect of serotonin, the symptoms are reversed.

Sumatriptan is only the first of what will be a whole series of even better serotonin-enhancing compounds. The molecular composition of these drugs will surprisingly be remarkably similar to several new compounds being developed to treat depression (although there is no statistical connection between migraines and depression, enhancing serotonin, such as the well-publicized drug Prozac does, is being shown to be an effective way of treating depression). The drugs will be injected to get them quickly into the bloodstream, and migraine patients will carry with them self-injectable, premeasured doses. Oral versions of the same drugs will be available for less severe migraines. By 1996, it will be possible for virtually one hundred percent relief from a migraine within thirty minutes after injection, an absolute godsend to millions.

## A PERFECT SMILE

Although we don't think of dentistry as a scientifically exciting branch of medicine, there is a great deal of research ongoing in the field using molecular biology, immunology and high-tech materials. In the next couple of decades this research is going to change our concept of dental care completely, as well as advance cosmetic dentistry to where results are not only perfect but far less expensive and available to most people.

It's been a long time since we've seen the old toothpaste commercials with the kids skipping home from the dentist joyously proclaiming, "Look, Ma, no cavities!" Our perception is that dental caries is no longer a problem for either children or adults.

This isn't true. Children are still getting cavities, although they get them less often and later in life—50 percent of seventeen-year-olds now compared with 90 percent of preteenagers thirty years ago. Adults still develop dental caries, too. Fluoride in toothpaste and the water supply is generally given credit by dental authorities for what improvements we have seen, but we need to do better. Fluoride has not been completely effective. It only works on certain kinds of cavities. In addition, some recent laboratory studies show that high levels of fluoride are toxic to animals, adding fuel to the often emotionally charged, irrational arguments of fluoridation opponents.

We are going to have a more effective measure than fluoride, and relatively soon. For the past several years researchers have been studying a vaccine to prevent cavities. The vaccine leads to the production by our immune system of antibodies against a bacterium called *Streptococcus mutans*, the organism chiefly responsible for cavities and a relative of the bug that causes strep throats. It has already been shown to be 85 percent effective. Until recently, however, there wasn't much hope for this vaccine because the antibodies against this organism cross-react with heart tissue, potentially leading to a pathology similar to that of rheumatic fever.

Bioengineering has solved this problem. By using a methodology called recombinant technology to purify the vaccine material, the antibodies our immune system produces are highly specific and react only with the *Streptococcus* organism. All cross-reactivity—and therefore the danger—has been eliminated. Tests are beginning now, and by the year 2000, all children will be vaccinated against cavities, a method that will be virtually 100 percent effective.

More research is being devoted to the number one dental problem of today—periodontal disease, the loss of bone that supports our gums and teeth. Although great progress is being made, even to the point where within fifteen to twenty years flossing to save our teeth may become unnecessary, periodontal disease is much more complicated then caries. Therefore, several solutions are being pursued.

As with cavities, researchers are looking at bacteria in the mouth as an important cause of the disease, and this will eventually lead to a vaccine. But whereas there is only one type of organism associated with caries, with periodontal problems there are at least four. It hasn't yet been determined if it is necessary to immunize against all of these bacteria to protect against development of periodontal disease. In a special type of periodontal disease, juvenile periodontitis, there is only one bacterium involved which causes rapid bone loss. This may prove to be the case with ordinary periodontal disease as well. If so, developing a vaccine will be much easier and we could see it by the year 2000. Otherwise, it will be necessary to use genetic engineering to develop a polyvalent vaccine—one that immunizes against more than one type of bacteria—and that will take up to twenty years.

In the meantime, research is going ahead full force in treatment of periodontal disease. Nonsteriod antiinflammatory drugs (relatives of the common over-the-counter drug ibuprofen) have been shown in both tissue culture and laboratory animals to inhibit bone loss. Now human clinical trials are about to begin with bioengineered derivatives that should work more specifically and effectively than ibuprofen. We should see these drugs used within five years to help stop bone loss at an early stage and make most surgery unnecessary.

Used in conjunction with the antiinflammatory drugs will be techniques to build back the bone. In the next ten years, periodontists will transplant bone from one part of the body to the mouth, and sometimes incorporate it with sturdy, innovative artificial materials. By about 2006, the hottest, most exciting area of current periodontal research will be routinely applied, the use of growth factors to stimulate new bone growth in the mouth. These are molecular variants of the compounds used to encourage regeneration of brain and nerve cells. By 2010, these growth factors and the preventive vaccines will be the mainstays of what will completely eliminate the need for surgery and will eventually wipe out periodontal disease completely.

## THROW AWAY YOUR EYEGLASSES— AND ADJUST YOUR EYES

Since more than half of all of us wear corrective lenses of some kind, visual problems can't be considered abnormal. Still, if given our choice, most of us would prefer not to wear glasses or to have to fumble every day with contact lenses. And we'd also certainly rather not have to adjust to using bifocals as we get older.

Opticians aren't about to go out of business completely, but for about 75 percent of us—those whose nearsightedness or farsightedness isn't too severe—there will be no need to wear corrective lenses. Instead of periodically visiting our optician or optometrist to have our prescription for glasses or contact lenses adjusted, we're going to visit our ophthalmologist to have our *eyes* adjusted.

Using a relatively new type of laser called an ultraviolet excimer, ophthalmologists, first at the Charlottenburg Clinic in Berlin, Germany, and subsequently at several other facilities around the world, have successfully corrected nearsightedness by "sculpturing" the eyes. Most visual problems come because the cornea, the thin outer covering of our eyes, changes shape as we develop from early childhood. If it becomes too convex the result is nearsightedness; too much concavity causes farsightedness. The excimer lasers are so accurate and precise they can vaporize layers of the cornea less than a millionth of an inch thick, flattening it to treat nearsighted patients and making it rounder to correct farsightedness. The entire procedure takes just a few seconds.

For now, the technique remains experimental, as not enough experience has been gained to predict the degree of correction the procedure will provide. Undershooting could be corrected by an additional procedure, but overshooting would be more difficult to remedy. In addition, a small percentage of patients have complained about eye pain and a filmy sensation. Although both side effects were temporary and gone within a few days, ophthalmologists aren't ready to rush in with eye sculpturing. It won't be used until it's perfect. That won't take very long, however. By 1997, ophthalmologists around the world will have gained enough experience to routinely use eye sculpturing, and laser development will keep pace, making the procedure even more precise.

—— SHRINK YOUR PROSTATE, GROW YOUR HAIR ——

When we're very young, every part of our body still seems to be the right size and in the right place. But as we get older, no matter how how hard we battle, things change. We gain and lose in the places where we can least afford to do either. For me, there's no better example than our head and our prostate gland. Most of us seem to exchange a full head of hair and a small prostate for at least partial baldness and an enlarged prostate, one that presses on our urinary outlet like a clamp on a garden hose and forces us out of sleep to the bathroom at least once a night.

But why discuss baldness and an enlarged prostate together? These are only two signs of aging. Surely they can't be connected.

In fact, while they are not actually connected, there is a similar biochemical process responsible for both occurrences, and there will be similar biochemical treatments.

There are no known medical consequences of baldness, aside from some scalp sunburn and a bruised ego, so prostate enlargement—which can cause urinary retention and kidney infections—has been attacked first. We've already heard about the drugs to shrink enlarged prostates. The first ones introduced are called finasteride (named Proscar by its manufacturer) and terazosin (trade name Hytrin). In large clinical trials, both of them reduced prostate size by at least 20 percent in more than half of the patients treated and produced continuous improvement in urine flow in almost 60 percent. With more progress in formulating these drugs and the eventual use of them preventively, the results will be even better. By the turn of the century, most of the hundreds of thousands of operations performed every year to either shrink the prostate or remove it completely will be unnecessary.

The prostate-shrinking drugs belong to a class of compounds known as 5-alpha-reductase inhibitors. They block the key enzyme that converts the primary male sex hormone, testosterone, to a derivative called dihydrotestosterone or DHT. Among other things, DHT promotes the growth of the prostate.

Some of the "other things" that DHT is responsible for is where the connection between prostate enlargement and baldness lies. In the hair follicles of those who turn bald is an increased production of the enzyme that converts testosterone to DHT. When DHT is produced it acts on the follicle to slowly miniaturize it, and eventually it will no longer produce a hair shaft. Those follicles that don't make the enzyme continue to grow hair.

Understanding this process leaves scientists with a whole range of ways to molecularly manipulate hair growth, all of which will be far more effective then Rogaine, currently the only drug approved for treatment of baldness. Rogaine doesn't work at the molecular level at all, but only by increasing blood flow and skin temperature around the hair follicles.

We won't use exactly the same drugs as will be used to shrink or prevent enlarged prostates, but only slightly different formulations. Some will be applied topically, some we will take by mouth, others will be injectable. The first one will be available by mid-decade, a topically applied enzyme inhibitor. Since the hair follicles have only been dwarfed by DHT, not killed, they are capable of being rejuvenated. By applying this drug daily to thinning areas, the enzyme responsible for converting testosterone to DHT in the follicles will be blocked, and new hair shafts will sprout. It won't be just peach fuzz growth, as with Rogaine, but honest-to-goodness new hair.

A little further away, probably by 2001, we will take intervention one step earlier. As we know, most baldness is hereditary, carried in our genes. It's highly unlikely we'll ever see genetic therapy for baldness of the type we have discussed for the more serious diseases, i.e, the introduction of new genes. No matter what advances are made, genetic therapy will still be relatively complex treatment, and not entirely risk-free, pretty difficult to justify for baldness. But we will have the next best thing. The first drugs for baldness will inhibit the crucial enzyme after it's already produced. The later versions will stop the enzyme from ever being made.

The only disadvantage to either of these drugs is that it will need to be taken for a lifetime, or else the enzyme the genes have ordained in the follicle will begin to work again, testosterone will be converted again to DHT, and all the new hair we will have become so proud of will shrink away.

There is an ultimate solution, though. We've already seen how immunotherapy is going to be used in ways that we never dreamed, and here's another one. Men are going to be able to have vaccinations to prevent baldness. The injections will stimulate us to produce antibodies against the DHT and even eventually against the gene-regulating signals. Since these antibodies will circulate continuously in our bloodstream, we won't need to use inhibiting or regulating drugs daily. At worst, we might need an occasional baldness-fighting booster, a small inconvenience for a full head of hair.

## THE END OF BREAD-AND-BUTTER PATHOLOGY
## ———————— AND GALLSTONE SOUVENIRS ————————

Pathologists often describe the examination of gallbladders removed in surgery as bread-and-butter pathology. These are the routine and common specimens that can usually be diagnosed easily and quickly. Measure the gallbladder, open it, take a section for a microscopic slide to scrutinize tomorrow, count and measure the gallstones.

After the diagnosis has been made, the final step is often returning the stones to the patient. As bizarre as it may seem, I've often been told by operating room nurses that many people inlay tables with them; some even make necklaces. The cholesterol deposits that compose most gallstones do accrete in such a way that they can produce some interesting and, I suppose, beautiful patterns, similar to a South American fire opal. Even so, knowing the pathology that developed them and the pain they caused, I'd pass.

Soon, so will most everyone else. The treatment of gallstones is already undergoing some major changes, but this is just the beginning for millions of people. About 10 percent of the population in the Western world have gallstones. In the United States alone, a million new cases are diagnosed every year and 500,000 have their gallbladders removed because of intractable pain caused by the stones.

The surgical removal of the gallbladder (cholecystectomy) is usually a very safe procedure, but there is always a small risk associated with opening the abdominal cavity. Besides, surgery and hospitalization are expensive, and the recuperative period lasts several weeks. For these reasons, in the past few years there has been an explosion of alternatives to the bread-and-butter surgery.

The majority of gallbladders are now removed by video surgery, technically called laparoscopy. A few small needle-puncture incisions are made in the abdomen, and through them are inserted a video camera and the necessary surgical instruments. The gallbladder is set free from its abdominal moorings and removed through one of the tiny holes. The technique is cheaper. Patients are discharged the day after surgery (instead of three to five days later after a standard gallbladder surgery) and can return to work and even participate in sports within a week. Gallbladder surgery has become a minor procedure.

Although most surgeons feel laparoscopic surgery is being some-what oversold due to media and patient pressure, it is here to stay as a major surgical technique and will supplant old, painful open surgery as the treatment of choice for many conditions. With continued refinement of instruments and technique, it will soon be used to repair hernias, for appendectomies, even for some cancer surgery.

Even better than removing the gallbladder by laparoscopy will be laser surgery, a technique that we will see applied to gallstones before the end of the decade. Here, through the same type of incision now used to remove the gallbladder by laparoscopy, a camera-guided laser will be inserted into the bile ducts and, with a pulse of energy, will vaporize the stones.

Better medical treatments are on the horizon, too, not just to treat gallstones, but ultimately to prevent them from occurring in the first place. In the treatment area, gastroenterologists are continuing to make discoveries about the use of oral medication to dissolve gallstones. The bile acids currently being used have been modestly successful, but there is a high rate of recurrence of stones. The same can be said of electric shock wave therapy to fragment gallstones. Within the next five to seven years, we can expect advances with each of these modalities, especially oral bile acids, such that the number of gallbladders removed, even by video surgery, will be cut in half.

But the biggest advance is going to be a low-cost drug that will prevent gallstones by working at the most basic level where they are formed. It used to be thought that gallstones were simply the result of having too much cholesterol in the bile—something controlled by genetics and diet. But an additional factor is needed to cause the cholesterol to crystallize. This is called a nucleation factor, because it provides a nucleus around which the cholesterol can stratify over time in order to develop into a stone.

Several researchers are working on ways to attack the nucleation factors. One weapon is aspirin, that truly amazing drug for which we continue to find uses even after all these years. If prairie dogs (a curious experimental animal, but one whose metabolism is ideal for studying gallbladder pathology) are fed a high cholesterol diet, they make gallstones. But if they are fed aspirin along with the cholesterol, they don't make gallstones. Aspirin presumably works by modulating the synthesis of hormonelike substances called prostaglandins, which in turn inhibits the secretion of compounds called glycoproteins, thought to be nucleating factors for cholesterol gall-stones.

What works in prairie dogs, of course, doesn't necessarily work in humans, so this will have to be tested. It's unlikely aspirin is going to be the final word. Even more specific substances than aspirin will be found, and by the turn of the century we will have inexpensive and easy ways to administer antinucleating factors to prevent gallstones.

—— PREVENTING AND TREATING BRITTLE BONES ——

There are already more than 300,000 hip fractures a year in the United States from osteoporosis, and if present trends were allowed to continue, by 2020 the number would exceed 500,000. But this will not happen. It's taken some time, but researchers are finally making breakthroughs that will rapidly accelerate the diagnosis, treatment and prevention of osteoporosis. Instead of the number of hip fractures almost doubling by 2020, it actually will be reduced by at least 80 percent, as will the incidence of osteoporosis.

Some of the advances will begin to be applied in the next few years. Before the end of the decade, doctors will routinely measure bone mass right in their office as easily as they now take a blood pressure. The patients who have this test will initially all be women as they reach menopause. Once the genes that predispose to osteoporosis are identified, those who carry them will be tested as well. The test will be a noninvasive tool, will cost less than twenty dollars and will measure not only the density of the bone but the strength, something researchers now realize is at least as important as how much bone one has. It will be exquisitely predictive of future risk of osteoporosis.

Along with this ability to predict future risk are going to come dramatic developments in prevention and treatment, thanks to our ability to grow bone cells in a culture. Scientists are already able to scrutinize the laying down of bone and its resorption, a cycle that occurs continually in our bodies. Normally, the cells that lay down new bone (osteoblasts) work in synchrony with those that take away old bone (osteoclasts). However, in patients with osteoporosis, the process loses its harmony, and more bone is taken away than is laid down.

The best resorption preventive we have now is estrogen, although there have been some new drugs recently made available, calcitonin and biphosphonates. But estrogen is not the best-suited tool, because it may indeed increase the risk for breast cancer. Studies have been equivocal, but we will have a safe alternative before we have a definitive answer. A drug will be created by the computer modeling of the *interaction of estrogen* with its receptors on bone cells, so that it will be possible to isolate *just* the part of the molecule that is responsible for preventing bone loss. Based on this, a synthetic compound will be developed that is even more effective than estrogen alone and, even more important, has no effect at all on the breast.

The treatments of osteoporosis will be no less innovative. Presently the only drug that even remotely qualifies for the job is fluoride. But fluoride is largely unacceptable because it creates severe gastrointestinal side effects and because, although it does increase bone mass, it has no effect on bone quality. The new bone is no stronger.

But scientists have already come up with a far better alternative, one that will soon begin clinical testing. It involves just one molecular chip of a hormone produced by our parathyroid glands (four pea-sized fragments of tissue that sit in our neck on the four corners of our thyroid), which are the most important regulators of calcium metabolism and bone formation in our bodies. A synthetic version of this will be used routinely on patients by the end of the decade. It will be the first agent that actually improves both bone mass and quality. Then and only then will we be able to say that osteoporosis is reversible. Initially the drug will be given by injection, but eventually it will either be taken by a nasal spray or be coated so that it can be administered by mouth.

Further away, by 2010, we will see the manipulation of the actual control mechanisms that cause bone to be laid down and resorbed. Physicians will be able to manipulate this dynamic growth and resorption sequence by administering synthetic versions of the appropriate growth factors, causing new bone to be laid down more often than the old is taken away. It will be the most potent treatment we will develop, and even people severely crippled by osteoporosis will grow new bone and become mobile again.

## A NEW KIND OF ANTIBODY
### — TO TREAT DRUG OVERDOSES —

An automobile comes screeching up to the door of the busy city hospital emergency room, its horn blaring. A frantic father flies through the door carrying his limp, unconscious three-year-old child. As soon as the head nurse sees him, she snatches the child from his father's arms, signals the nearest doctor, and they rush into the largest, most fully equipped treatment room. They are moving so fast the child is practically thrown onto the gurney, the room suddenly awash in bright halogen and fluorescent lights and teeming with activity. The child's respiration is extremely shallow, barely perceptible; heart rate only 36; blood pressure way down, 60/40.

The father is so shaken he can barely speak, but while the doctor is checking the child's vital signs the nurse sees the father is holding an empty pill container in his right hand. She snatches it and reads the label: Percodan.

She grabs the father by the shoulders and pushes her face right into his. "How many did he swallow?" she demands. "And when?"

When he hesitates for a few seconds, the nurse shouts, "Tell me, damn it! We've only got a few minutes!"

"All of them, fourteen I think," answers the father, his voice trembling like Jell-O. "It must have been about an hour and a half ago."

While the physician inserts an intravenous line, the nurse rushes to the cabinet and pulls out a syringe marked: Percodan/pediatric.

"About thirty-five pounds," the nurse says, estimating the child's body weight.

"Push all of it," the doctor instructs her. And to another nurse, "Give me a laryngoscope with a pediatric blade and a number six endotracheal tube. His breathing is Cheyne-Stokes. In another minute, I'm gonna have to tube him. And get me a blood gas kit."

The nurse jams the needle into the rubber intravenous tubing and within five seconds pushes in the entire contents of the syringe.

"Is he gonna die?" The father can barely bite out the words, he's sobbing and shaking so much.

"Another fifteen, twenty minutes, he would have for sure," answers the doctor without looking up. "But we may have got him in time. We'll know more in just a few minutes."

Despite his protestations, the nurse ushers the father out of the treatment room, where he is comforted briefly by another nurse on her way to assist with a stab wound.

His agony is not prolonged. Within five minutes the child's heart rate has risen to 65, the blood pressure to 80/50, the respirations are regular and deep. The child starts to cry. So does his father.

"He'll have to stay with us a few days, but he's going to be all right, thank God," says the nurse.

This miracle is taking place in 1998. The syringe the nurse used was a computer-designed substance called a catalytic antibody. It is a hybrid of a specific antibody against a specific drug. It was developed through bioengineering, and then it was chemically bound to an enzyme that rapidly breaks down the drug. It is an advance over even monoclonal antibodies in that it not only is specific for a particular substance, but binds to only one site on that substance, the site where the enzyme brought along for the ride can immediately break down the drug.

In the drug cabinet of every hospital emergency room is a whole array of color-coded syringes, each for a specific drug. Although not every drug in the *Physician's Desk Reference* is represented, more then twenty-five of the most common substances, both street drugs and prescription medications, are covered. An overdose can be treated effectively and completely within minutes. The death rate has dropped dramatically.

By 2008, these coded syringes will have proven so effective that rapidly absorbable subcutaneous versions, which can be easily administered by anyone, will have been created. This will allow any parents with small children to purchase the specific catalytic antibody syringe to have on hand whenever they buy a potentially dangerous drug. Such syringes, will also be distributed free to the mates and friends of street drug addicts and, until we solve the drug problem with molecular prevention, will save countless thousands more lives.

And the miracle making will continue.

# Epilogue

THE OVERWHELMING BULK OF EVIDENCE IN THIS BOOK MUST FI-
nally give rise to an optimism about the future. But do not think
you are seeing Utopia. There are paradoxes and contradictions
in this picture. And it is still going to be the rich who will benefit the most, although inevitably we will see some benefits for
the poor—even as the gap between rich and poor continues to
widen.

The most worrisome possibility for a dark side is directly related to the amazing ability we are going to have to predict an individual's future predisposition to disease at or before birth. The
trouble is that the information we will be able to gather could be
used for purposes other than prevention. The crucial issue will be
privacy.

Even though predictive technology is still in its infancy, terms
such as "genetically unemployable" and "genetically uninsurable"
are already creeping into our vocabulary. Will the results of these
predictive profiles—available at birth—be held private or will insurance companies and employers have access to them? And what
will they do with this information—what will they be allowed to

do—if it is made more public? Will an insurance company be permitted to refuse coverage, or to require lifetime higher premiums, for a newborn with a genetic susceptibility to cancer or to Alzheimer's disease? And will we consider it correct for a potential employer, such as an airline, to reject a perfectly healthy applicant for a pilot's job because of a higher than normal risk for heart disease? Since this determination would have been made at birth, should this person have been prevented from becoming a pilot in the first place?

Knowing that such information could be used against them, will some parents be deterred from having such tests performed on their newborns, denying their children an awareness of a disease predisposition that could be corrected by the new preventive technology? Or will there be no choice? Perhaps it will be required by law that these tests be routinely performed on all newborns. Will this lead to a new form of eugenics?

Why, you might ask, would insurance companies be inclined to deny coverage to someone who was born with a genetic predisposition to a disease? Haven't we just depicted a scenario in which, with just a few turns of a molecular wrench, that predisposition can be eliminated? The answer is yes. But there will be a gap—a period of about ten to fifteen years between our ability to predict and our ability to alter.

This prediction-prevention gap creates another issue. Results of DNA tests will be helpful only if something can be done about them. Knowing that someone has inherited a susceptibility to heart disease or a certain type of cancer will allow us to begin whatever methods of prevention are currently available. But what if the news is that one's baby has inherited the genes for a disease for which we are still years away from a deterrent or reversal? And what if we find this out long enough before birth to stop the process? Another agony of choice begins.

And how will we exercise our options when it becomes possible to predict predisposition not only to disease but to intelligence, athletic ability and creativity as well? Used properly, knowing that one's newborn has inherited a special talent or capability could be a blessing. Right from the start, an environment could be provided that would best nurture and foster the development of what the genes have given.

Used improperly, however, this information could be a mixed

blessing, or worse. Instead of providing an environment in which a child's special talents would be allowed to flower, we might see the ultimate Little League syndrome develop. Parents could be tempted to put tremendous psychological pressure on their children, accusing them of not trying hard enough, not living up to their genes. In addition, the temptation could be great to create one-dimensional children. Why should Johnny waste time playing the guitar when his genetic profile says his strongest abilities lie in mathematics? The fact that Johnny might actually enjoy the guitar, even though he may never be great at it, should count for something in the society of the future. And what about the child whose genes indicate intellectual inferiority? Will that child be deprived of love and nurturing because his parents have given up on him?

When it finally becomes possible to actually change one's inherited abilities, will this alteration qualify as medical therapy? Will the doctors specializing in enhancement therapy be the future and ultimate version of today's cosmetic surgeons? Will we be able to afford to indulge in these procedures?

Although most of the tools for changing a predisposition to disease will make medical care cheaper and will eventually be available to everyone, enhancement tools will not. They will be costly, and insurance will not pay for them. Genetic enhancement will be an option for the wealthy only. Although society already tolerates certain inequities between the haves and the have-nots, we are going to have to decide how far we are willing to let this go. Having the means to send one's children to private school is one thing, but being able to molecularly alter their intelligence or athletic ability is another.

Researchers are well aware of the potential harm that could be caused by misinterpretation or misuse of genetic profiles, and are calling for intensive training of genetic counselors whose guidance will accompany any results. And, in an unprecedented move, commensurate with the unprecedented nature of its scientific endeavor, the Human Genome Project has set aside 3 percent of its funding for ethical considerations.

Our fear of technology is not about to quickly abate, nor will our current unhappiness with medical care vanish overnight. But nonetheless, we have to be enormously encouraged. The fact remains that millions of people are going to be the direct beneficiaries of fundamental changes that will bring blessed relief to those afflicted with diseases for which there are presently no cures or prevention. We will understand that medical research, in its own peculiar way, always stumbles forward, looking for a cure to one disease, and suddenly finding a solution to another along the way. Our destiny is not doom.

Our destiny is to make things better.

# Note of Appreciation

WRITING A BOOK IS BY NATURE SOLITARY. SEVERAL PEOPLE HAVE made this one much less so.

I thank my literary agents, Herb and Nancy Katz, who are not just my agents, but friends and confidants.

I am grateful to my editor at Simon & Schuster, Fred Hills, for immediately seeing the value of *Rx 2000* and championing it throughout, to his colleague Daphne Bien, who is a careful and alert reader, and also to Phil James, for his astute copy editing.

I thank Howard Edsall, who has freely and frequently benefitted me with his journalistic advice and support, honed by more than fifty years at the typewriter. I also thank Sara Gusik, my research assistant, for so promptly finding and delivering the hundreds of scientific articles I requested.

I thank my wife, Liz, a.k.a. superwoman, who, despite starting her own business while I was writing this book, was there for me always, providing comfort, love, reassurance, running companionship, a sympathetic ear and even dinner (as long as I did the dishes). I hope I haven't been too absorbed to let her know how much I love her.

229

# Bibliography

——— INTRODUCTION: AN INTIMATE TECHNOLOGY ———

Antonarkis SE.   Diagnosis of genetic disorders at the DNA level. *New England Journal of Medicine* 1989; 320:153–163.

Goodridge AG.   The new metabolism: molecular genetics in the analysis of metabolic regulation. *Federation of American Societies for Experimental Biology Journal* 1990; 4:3099–3110.

Harper PS, Clarke A.   Should we test children for "adult" genetic diseases? *Lancet* 1990; 335:1205–1206.

Landegren U, Kaiser R, Caskey CT, Hood LH.   DNA diagnosis—molecular techniques and automation. *Science* 1988; 242:229–237.

McKusick VA.   Current trends in mapping human genes. *Federation of American Societies for Experimental Biology Journal* 1991; 5:12–20.

Rossiter BJF, Caskey CT.   Molecular studies of human genetic disease. *Federation of American Societies for Experimental Biology Journal* 1991; 5:21–27.

Watson JD.   The human genome project: past, present and future. *Science* 1990; 248:44–49.

Watson JD, Crick FHC.   Molecular structure of nucleic acids: a structure of deoxyribose nucleic acid. *Nature* 1953; 171:737–738.

CHAPTER 1:
- THE ULTIMATE SEPARATION OF SEX AND REPRODUCTION -

Aitken J.   Do sperm find eggs attractive? *Nature* 1991; 351(2):19–20.

Barker PE.   Gene mapping and cystic fibrosis. *American Journal of Medical Science* 1990; 299:69–72.

Bouchard TJ, Jr, Lykken DT, McGue, et al.   Sources of human psychological differences: the Minnesota study of twins reared apart. *Science* 1990; 250:223–228.

Cohen J, Adler A, Alikani M, et al.   Partial zona dissection or subzonal sperm insertion: microsurgical fertilization alternatives based on evaluation of sperm and embryo morphology. *Fertility and Sterility* 1991; 56(4):696–706.

Garrisi GJ, Talansky BE, Grunfeld L, et al.   Clinical evaluation of three approaches to micromanipulation-assisted fertilization. *Fertility and Sterility* 1990; 54(4):671–677.

Levran D, Dor J, Rudak E, et al.   Pregnancy potential of human oocytes—the effect of cryopreservation. *New England Journal of Medicine* 1990; 323:1153–1156.

Lubin, MB, Lin HJ, Vadheim CM, Rotter JI.   Genetics of common diseases of adulthood: implications for prenatal counseling and diagnosis. *Clinics in Perinatology* 1990; 17:889–910.

Malhstedt PP, Probasco KA.   Sperm donors: their attitudes toward providing medical and psychosocial information for recipient couples and donor offspring. *Fertility and Sterility* 1991; 56(4):747–753.

Meissen GJ, Myers RH, Mastromauro CA, et al.   Predictive testing for Huntington's disease with use of a linked DNA marker. *New England Journal of Medicine* 1988; 318:535–542.

Mullis K, Faloona F, Scharf S, et al.   Specific enzymatic amplification of DNA in vitro: the polymerase chain reaction. *Cold Spring Harbor Symposium in Quantitative Biology* 1986; 51:263–273.

Rommens JM, Iannuzzi MC, Kerem B-S, et al.   Identification of the cystic fibrosis gene: chromosome walking and jumping. *Science* 1989; 245:1059–1065.

Rose EA.   Applications of the polymerase chain reaction to genome analysis. *Federation of American Societies for Experimental Biology Journal* 1991; 5:56–63.

Rossiter BJF, Caskey CT.   Molecular studies of human genetic disease. *Federation of American Societies for Experimental Biology Journal* 1991; 5:21–27.

Sauer MV, Paulson RJ, Lobo R.   A preliminary report on oocyte donation extending reproductive potential to women over 40. *New England Journal of Medicine* 1990; 323:1157–1160.

Wright PA, Wynford-Thomas D.   The polymerase chain reaction: miracle or mirage? a critical review of its uses and limitations in diagnosis and research. *Journal of Pathology* 1990; 162:99–117.


———————— CHAPTER 2: THE GARDENING OF THE BODY ————————

Davis RB III, Schneck DJ.  A fluid mechanics approach to the problem of sensory feedback in prosthetic devices. In Schneck DF (editor): *Biofluid Mechanics*, vol 2. New York (1980), Plenum Press, 147–160.

Francione GL.  Xenografts and animal rights. *Transplantation Proceedings* 1990; 22(3):1044–1046.

Khouri RK, Koudsi B, Reddi H.  Tissue transformation into bone in vivo. *Journal of the American Medical Association* 1991; 266(14):1953–1955.

Macleod AM, Thomson AW.  FK 506: an immunosuppressant for the 1990s? *Lancet* 1991; 337:25–27.

Mikulecky DC, Clarke AM (editors).  *Biomedical Engineering: Opening New Doors*. New York (1990), New York University Press.

Randall T.  New antirejection drug anticipated. *Journal of the American Medical Association* 1990; 264(10):1225–1226.

Reemtsma K.  Ethical aspects of xenotransplantation. *Transplantation Proceedings* 1990; 22(3):1042–1043.

Sachs DH.  Antigen-specific transplantion tolerance. *Clinical Transplantation* 1990; 4:78–81.

Sachs DH, Sharabi Y, Sykes M.  Mixed chimerism and transplantation tolerance. *Progress in Immunology* 1989; 7:1171–1176.

Schneck, DJ.  *Engineering Principles of Physiologic Function*. New York (1990), New York University Press.

Singer PA.  A review of public policies to procure and distribute kidneys for transplantation. *Archives of Internal Medicine* 1990; 150:523–527.

Starzl TE, Fung J, Jordan M, et al.  Kidney transplantation under FK 506. *Journal of the American Medical Association* 1990; 264:63–67.

Sternberg H, Segall PE, Waitz H, Ben-Abraham A.  Interventive gerontology, cloning and cryonics: relevance to life extension. In *Biomedical Advances in Aging*. New York (1990), Plenum Press, 207–219.

Wight JP.  Ethics, commerce and kidneys. *British Medical Journal* 1991; 303:110.


———————— CHAPTER 3: OUTTHINKING THE BRAIN ————————

Blum K, Noble EP, Sheridan PJ, et al.  Allelic association of human dopamine, $D_2$ receptor gene in alcoholism. *Journal of the American Medical Association* 1990; 263:2055–2060.

Bray GA.   Treatment for obesity: a nutrient balance/nutrient partition approach. *Nutrition Reviews* 1991; 49(2):33–45.

Comings DE, Comings BF, Muhleman D, et al.   The dopamine $D_2$ receptor locus as a modifying gene in neuropsychiatric disorders. *Journal of the American Medical Association* 1991; 266:1793–1800.

Marx J.   Marijuana receptor gene cloned. *Science* 1990; 249:624–626.

Noble EP, Blum K.   The dopamine $D_2$ receptor gene and alcoholism. *Journal of the American Medical Association* 1991; 265:2667.

Noble EP, Blum K, Ritchie T, et al.   Allelic association of the $D_2$ dopamine receptor gene with receptor binding characteristics in alcoholism. *Archives of General Psychiatry* 1991; 48:648–654.

Snyder SH.   Planning for serendipity. *Nature* 1990; 346:508.

Trujillo KA, Akil H.   Inhibition of morphine tolerance and dependence by the NMDA receptor antagonist MK-801. *Science* 1991; 251:85–87.

## CHAPTER 4:
### —————— THE HOSPITAL IN YOUR LIVING ROOM ——————

Allison AC, Gregoriadis G.   Vaccines: recent trends and progress. *Immunology Today* 1990; 11(12)427–429.

Eddy DM.   Connecting value and costs: whom do we ask and what do we ask them? *Journal of the American Medical Association* 1990; 264(13):1737–1739.

Eddy DM.   What care is essential? What services are basic? *Journal of the American Medical Association* 1991; 265(6):782–788.

Eddy DM.   What do we do about costs? *Journal of the American Medical Association* 1990; 264(9):1161–1170.

Grundy SM.   Recent nutrition research: implications for foods of the future. *Annals of Medicine* 1991; 23(2):187–193

Lundberg GD.   The direct access pathology laboratory. *American Society of Clinical Pathology News,* May/June 1990.

Soloway HB.   Patient-initiated laboratory testing: applauding the inevitable. *Journal of the American Medical Association* 1990; 264:1718–1719.

### —————— CHAPTER 5: THE TIMING OF OUR LIVES ——————

Badwe RA, Gregory WM, Chaudary MA, et al.   Timing of surgery during menstrual cycle and survival of premenopausal women with operable breast cancer. *Lancet* 1991; 337:1261–1264.

Czeisler CA, Johnson MP, Duffy JF, et al.   Exposure to bright light and darkness to treat physiologic maladaption to night work. *New England Journal of Medicine* 1990; 322:1253–1259.

Hrushesky WJM. More evidence for circadian rhythm effects in cancer chemotherapy: the fluorpyrimidine story. *Cancer Cells* 1990; 2(3):65–68.

Hrushesky WJM, Bluming AZ, Gruber SA, Sothern RB. Menstrual influence on surgical cure of breast cancer. *Lancet* 1989; 335:949–952.

Hrushesky WJM, Fader D, Schmitt O, Gilbertsen V. The respiratory sinus arrhythmia: a measure of cardiac age. *Science* 1984; 224:1001–1004.

Lemmer B (editor). *Chronopharmacology: Cellular and Biochemical Interactions.* New York and Basel (1989) Marcel Dekker, Inc., 439–473.

Moore-Ede M, Czeisler CA, Richardson GS. Circadian timekeeping in health and disease. Part 1: Basic principles of circadian pacemakers. *New England Journal of Medicine* 1983; 309(8):469–476.

Moore-Ede M, Czeisler CA, Richardson GS. Circadian timekeeping in health and disease. Part 2: Clinical implications of circadian rhythmicity. *New England Journal of Medicine* 1983; 309(9):530–536.

Moore-Ede M, Richardson GS. Medical implications of shift work. *Annual Review of Medicine* 1985; 36:607–617.

Panza JA, Epstein SE, Quyyumi AA. Circadian variation in vascular tone and its relation to a-sympathetic vasoconstrictor activity. *New England Journal of Medicine* 1991; 325:986–990.

Pepine CJ. Circadian variations in myocardial ischemia: implications for management. *Journal of the American Medical Association* 1991; 265:386–390.

Quyyumi AA. Circadian rhythms in cardiovascular disease. *American Heart Journal* 1990; 120:726–733.

Senie RT, Rosen PP, Rhodes P, Lesser ML. Timing of breast cancer excision influences duration of disease-free survival. *Annals of Internal Medicine* 1991; 115(5):337–342.

Thompson C, Stinson D, Smith A. Seasonal affective disorder and season-dependent abnormalities of melatonin suppression by light. *Lancet* 1990; 336:703–706.

---

## TIMELINE

Albert MB, Fromm H, Borstelmann R, et al. Successful outpatient treatment of gallstones with piezoelectric lithotripsy. *Annals of Internal Medicine* 1990; 113(2):164–166.

Anand R, Wesnes KA. Moclobemide, a reversible MAO inhibitor possesses cognition enhancing effects in humans. *Acta Psychiatrica Scandinavica Supplement* 1990; 82/360:71–72.

Andrews L, Jaeger A. Confidentiality of genetic information in the workplace. *American Journal of Law and Medicine* 1991; 17:75–108.

Arend W, Dayer J-M. Cytokines and cytokine inhibitors or antagonists in rheumatoid arthritis. *Arthritis and Rheumatism* 1990; 33(3):305–315.

Austin MA, King M-C, Vranizan KM, Kraus RM. Atherogenic lipoprotein phenotype: a proposed genetic marker for coronary heart disease risk. *Circulation* 1990; 82:495–506.

Barker PE. Gene mapping and cystic fibrosis. *American Journal of Medical Science* 1990; 299:69–72.

Baulieu E-E. Editorial: RU-486 and the early nineties. *Endocrinology* 1990; 127(5):2043–2046.

Blum K, Noble EP, Sheridan PJ, et al. Allelic association of human dopamine $D_2$ receptor gene in alcoholism. *Journal of the American Medical Association* 1990; 263:2055–2060.

Bolognesi DP. AIDS vaccines: progress and unmet challenges. *Annals of Internal Medicine* 1991; 114(2):161–162.

Bray GA. Treatment for obesity: a nutrient balance/nutrient partition approach. *Nutrition Reviews* 1991; 49(2):33–45.

Breslow JL. Genetic basis of lipoprotein disorders. *Journal of Clinical Investigation* 1989; 84:373–380.

Broder S (moderator). Antiretroviral therapy in AIDS. *Annals of Internal Medicine* 1990; 113(8):604–618.

Bruckstein AH. Nonsurgical management of cholelithiasis. *Archives of Internal Medicine* 1990; 150:960–964.

Cady RK, Wendt JK, Kirchner JR, et al. Treatment of acute migraine with subcutaneous sumatriptan. *Journal of the American Medical Association* 1991; 265:2831–2835.

Canalis E, McCarthy TL, Centrella M. Growth factors and cytokines in bone cell metabolism. *Annual Review of Medicine* 1991; 42:17–24.

Cannon GW, Emkey RD, Denes A, et al. Prospective two-year followup of recombinant interferon-γ in rheumatoid arthritis. *Journal of Rheumatology* 1990; 17:304–310.

Catalona WJ, Smith DS, Ratliff TL, et al. Measurement of prostate-specific antigen in serum as a screening test for prostate cancer. *New England Journal of Medicine* 1991; 324:1156–1161.

Charney DS, Krystal JH, Delgado PL, Heninger GR. Serotonin-specific drugs for anxiety and depressive disorders. *Annual Review of Medicine* 1990; 41:437–446.

Christiansen C. Consensus development conference: prophylaxis and treatment of osteoporosis. *American Journal of Medicine* 1991; 90:107–110.

Ciaranello RD, Ciaranello AL. Genetics of major psychiatric disorders. *Annual Review of Medicine* 1991; 42:151–158.

Comings DE, Comings BF, Muhleman D, et al. The dopamine $D_2$ receptor locus as a modifying gene in neuropsychiatric disorders. *Journal of the American Medical Association* 1991; 266:1793–1800.

Council on Ethical and Judicial Affairs, American Medical Association. Use of genetic testing by employers. *Journal of the American Medical Association* 1991; 266:1827–1830.

Culliton BJ. Gene therapy: into the home stretch. *Science* 1990; 249:974–976.

Czeisler CA, Johnson MP, Duffy JF, et al. Exposure to bright light and darkness to treat physiologic maladaption to nightwork. *New England Journal of Medicine* 1990; 322:1253–1259.

Davies TF, Martin A, Concepion ES, et al. Evidence of limited variability of antigent receptors on intrathyroidal T cells in autoimmune thyroid disease. *New England Journal of Medicine* 1991; 325:238–244.

Davis RE, Moos WH. Cholinergic replacement in dementia: past and future perspectives. *Clinical Advancements in Alzheimer's disease, in press.*

Dean M, Gerrard B, Steward C, et al. Identification of cystic fibrosis mutations. *Advances in Experimental Medicine and Biology* 1991; 290:45–51.

Djerassi C. Fertility awareness: jet-age rhythm method? *Science* 1990; 248:1061–1062.

Eddy DM. Connecting value and costs: whom do we ask and what do we ask them? *Journal of the American Medical Association* 1990; 264(13):1737–1739.

Eddy DM. What care is essential? What services are basic? *Journal of the American Medical Association* 1991; 265(6):782–788.

Eddy DM. What do we do about costs? *Journal of the American Medical Association* 1990; 264(9):1161–1170.

Editorial. Acetylcysteine. *Lancet* 1991; 337:1069–1070.

Enthoven A, Kronick R. A consumer-choice health plan for the 1990s. *New England Journal of Medicine* 1989; 320(2):29–37, 94–101.

Erickson D. Love and terror: is a chemical messenger key to treating Alzheimer's? *Scientific American* 1991; April:148–150.

Feigner PL, Rhodes G. Gene therapeutics. *Nature* 1991; 349:351–352.

Ferrari, MD, et al. (The Subcutaneous Sumatriptan International Study Group). Treatment of migraine attacks with sumatriptan. *New England Journal of Medicine* 1991; 325:316–321.

Fiatarone MA, Marks EC, Ryan N, et al. High-intensity strength training in nonagenarians. *Journal of the American Medical Association* 1990; 263:3029–3034.

Fikrig E, Barthold SW, Kantor FS, Flavell RA. Protection of mice against the lyme disease agent with recombinant OspA. *Science* 1990; 250:553–556.

Gage FH, Kawaja MD, Fisher LJ. Genetically modifed cells: applications for intracerebral grafting. *Trends in Neurosciences* 1991; 14(8):328–333.

Garrisi GJ, Talansky BE, Grunfeld L, et al. Clinical evaluation of three approaches to micromanipulation-assisted fertilization. *Fertility and Sterility* 1990; 54(4):671–677.

Goate AM, Haynes AR, Owen MJ, et al. Predisposing locus for Alzheimer's disease on chromosome 21. *Lancet* 1989; II:352–355.

Gold D, Bowden R, Sixbey J, et al. Chronic fatigue: a prospective clinical and virologic study. *Journal of the American Medical Association* 1990; 264:48–53.

Goldsmith M. Future surgery: minimal invasion. *Journal of the American Medical Association* 1990; 262(21):2723.

Goldsmith MA. From molecular biology to "genetic antibiotics." *Perspectives in Biology and Medicine* 1990; 34(1):99–108.

Gostin L. Genetic discrimination: the use of genetically based diagnostic and prognostic tests by employers and insurers. *American Journal of Law and Medicine* 1991; 17:109–144.

Goy J-J, Sigwart U, Vogt P, et al. Long-term follow-up of the first 56 patients treated with intracoronary self-expanding stents (the Lausanne experience). *American Journal of Cardiology* 1991; 67:569–572.

Grundy SM. Cholesterol and coronary heart disease: future directions. *Journal of the American Medical Association* 1990; 264(23):3053–3059.

Gunby P. "Decade of Brain'" holds promise for answers to schizophrenia. *Journal of the American Medical Association* 1990; 264(19):2483.

Harris WH, Sledge CB. Total hip and knee replacement. (First of two parts.) *New England Journal of Medicine* 1990; 323(11):725–731.

Harris WH, Sledge CB. Total hip and knee replacement. (Second of two parts.) *New England Journal of Medicine* 1990; 323(12):801–807.

Heaney RP, Avioli LV, Chestnut C III, et al. Osteoporotic bone fragility: detection by ultrasound transmission velocity. *Journal of the American Medical Association* 1989; 261:2986–2990.

Hess E. Cytokine inhibitors and osteoarthritis. *Journal of Rheumatology* 1990; 17:1123–1124.

Hoffman AF. Nonsurgical treatment of gallstone disease. *Annual Review of Medicine* 1990; 41:401–415.

Hoffman EP, Brown RH, Jr, Kunkel LM. Dystrophin: the protein product of the Duchenne muscular dystrophy locus. *Cell* 1987; 51:919–928.

Hoffman M. New vector delivers genes to lung cells. *Science* 1991; 252:374.

Kerem B-T, Rommens JM, Buchanan JA, et al. Identification of the cystic fibrosis gene: genetic analysis. *Science* 1989; 245:1073–1080.

Kleinerman MJ. New pharmaceutical strategies devised in effort to treat schizophrenia effectively with less risk. *Journal of the American Medical Association* 1990; 264(19):2487.

Kuivaneimi H, Tromp G, Prockop DJ. Mutations in collagen genes: causes of rare and some common diseases in humans. *Federation of American Societies for Experimental Biology Journal* 1991; 5:2052–2060.

Leibowitz SF. The role of serotonin in eating disorders. *Drugs* 1990; 39(supplement 3):33–48.

Lerner RA, Benkovic SJ. Observations in the interface between immunology and chemistry. *Chemtracts—Organic Chemistry* 1990; 3:1–36.

Levran D, Dor J, Rudak E, et al. Pregnancy potential of human oocytes—the effect of cryopreservation. *New England Journal of Medicine* 1990; 323:1153–1156.

Lindsay R. Managing osteoporosis: current trends, future possibilities. *Geriatrics* 1987; 42(3):35–39.

Litvack F, Eigler NL, Margolis JR, et al. Percutaneous excimer laser coronary angioplasty. *American Journal of Cardiology* 1990; 66:1027–1030.

Longaker MT, Golbus MS, Filly RA, et al. Maternal outcome after open fetal surgery. A review of the first 17 human cases. *Journal of the American Medical Association* 1991; 265:737–741.

Lundberg GD. The direct access pathology laboratory. *American Society of Clinical Pathology News*, May/June 1990.

Macleod AM, Thomson AW. FK 506: an immunosuppressant for the 1990s? *Lancet* 1991; 337:25–27.

Manning PJ, Watson RM, Margolskee DJ, et al. Inhibition of exercise-induced bronchoconstriction by MK-571, a potent leukotriene D4-receptor antagonist. *New England Journal of Medicine* 1990; 323:1736–1739.

Marx J. Gene identified for inherited cancer susceptibility. *Science* 1991; 253(5020):616.

Marx J. New clue to cancer metastasis found. *Science* 1990; 249:482–483.

Marx J. Testing of autoimmune therapy begins. *Science* 1991; 252:27–28.

Meyskens FL. Coming of age—the chemoprevention of cancer. *New England Journal of Medicine* 1990; 323:825–826.

Mitsuya H, Yarochoan R, Broder S. Molecular targets for AIDS therapy. *Science* 1990; 249:1533–1544.

Muller DWM, Ellis S, Debowey DL, Topol EJ. Quantitative angiographic comparison of the immediate success of coronary angioplasty, coronary atherectomy and endoluminal stenting. *American Journal of Cardiology* 1990; 66:938–942.

Nestel PJ. New lipoprotein profiles and coronary heart disease: improving precision of risk. *Circulation* 1990; 82(2):649–650.

Noble EP, Blum K. The dopamine $D_2$ receptor gene and alcoholism. *Journal of the American Medical Association* 1991; 265:2667.

Noble EP, Blum K, Ritchie T, et al. Allelic association of the $D_2$ dopamine receptor gene with receptor binding characteristics in alcoholism. *Archives of General Psychiatry* 1991; 48:648–654.

Orholm M, Munkholm P, Langholz E. Familial occurrence of inflammatory bowel disease. *New England Journal of Medicine* 1991; 324:84–88.

Palca J. Does a retrovirus explain fatigue syndrome puzzle? *Science* 1990; 249:1240–1241.

Partridge TA. Gene therapy: muscle transfection made easy. *Nature* 1991; 353(6338):757–758.

Paty DW, McFarlin DE, McDonald WI. Magnetic resonance imaging and laboratory aids in the diagnosis of multiple sclerosis. *Annals of Neurology* 1991; 29(1):3–5.

Peck WA, Riggs BL, Bell NH, et al. Research directions in osteoporosis. *American Journal of Medicine* 1988; 84:275–282.

Peshock RM. Clinical cardiovascular magnetic resonance imaging. *American Journal of Cardiology* 1990; 66:41F–44F.

Podolsky DK. Inflammatory bowel disease. *New England Journal of Medicine* 1991; 325(13):928–936.

Pool R. Making 3-D movies of the heart. *Science* 1991; 251:28–30.

Quinton PM. Cystic fibrosis: righting the wrong protein. *Nature* 1990; 347:226.

Raisz LG. Local and systemic factors in the pathogenesis of osteoporosis. *New England Journal of Medicine* 1988; 318(13):818–828.

Rajfer J, Aronson WJ, Bush PA, et al. Nitric oxide as a mediator of relaxation of the corpus cavernosum in response to nonadrenergic, noncholinergic neurotransmission. *New England Journal of Medicine* 1992; 326(2):90–94.

Randall T. Alzheimer's-linked protein found to be skin deep, but potential new therapies see beauty of it. *Journal of the American Medical Association* 1991; 265(3):309–310.

Randall T. New antirejection drugs anticipated. *Journal of the American Medical Association* 1990; 264(10):1225–1226.

Redfield RR, Birx DL, Ketter N, et al. A phase I evaluation of the safety and immunogenicity of vaccination with recombinant gp160 in patients with early human immunodeficiency virus infection. *New England Journal of Medicine* 1991; 324:1677–1684.

Reichel W, Dyck AJ. Euthanasia: a contemporary moral quandary. *Lancet* 1989; 334:1321–1324.

Richelson E. Antidepressants and brain neurochemistry. *Mayo Clinic Proceedings* 1990; 65:1227–1236.

Riordan JR, Alon N, Grzelczak Z, et al. The CF gene product as a member of a membrane transporter super family. *Advances in Experimental Medicine and Biology* 1991; 290:19–29.

Roberts L. Testing for cancer risk: tough questions ahead. *Science* 1991; 253(5020):614–615.

Rommens JM, Iannuzzi MC, Kerem B-S, et al. Identification of the cystic fibrosis gene: chromosome walking and jumping. *Science* 1989; 245:1059–1065.

Rosenberg SA, Aebersold P, Cornetta K, et al. Gene transfer into humans—immunotherapy of patients with advanced melanoma, using tumor-infiltrating lymphocytes modified by retroviral gene transduction. *New England Journal of Medicine* 1990; 323:570–578.

Sachs DH. Antigen-specific transplantion tolerance. *Clinical Transplantation* 1990; 4:78–81.

Sachs DH, Sharabi Y, Sykes M. Mixed chimerism and transplantation tolerance. *Progress in Immunology* 1989; 7:1171–1176.

Safian RD, Gelbfish JS, Erny RE, et al. Coronary atherectomy: clinical, angiographic and histological findings and observations regarding potential mechanisms. *Circulation* 1990; 82:69–79.

Sauer MV, Paulson RJ, Lobo R. A preliminary report on oocyte donation extending reproductive potential to women over 40. *New England Journal of Medicine* 1990; 323:1157–1160.

Schoenfield LJ, Berci G, Carnovale RL, et al. The effect of ursodial on the efficacy and safety of extracorporeal shock-wave lithotripsy of gallstones. *New England Journal of Medicine* 1990; 323:1239–1245.

Selkoe D. Deciphering Alzheimer's disease: the amyloid precursor protein yields new clues. *Science* 1990; 248:1058–1060.

Sennhauser FH, Liechti-Gallati S, Moser H. Screening for carriers of cystic fibrosis among partners of people heterozygous for the disease. *British Medical Journal* 1990; 301:1081.

Shields PG, Harris CC. Molecular epidemiology and the genetics of environmental cancer. *Journal of the American Medical Association* 1991; 266:681–687.

Sidransky D, Eschenbach A, Tsai YC, et al. Identification of p53 gene mutations in bladder cancers and urine samples. *Science* 1991; 252:706–709.

Singer PA. A review of public policies to procure and distribute kidneys for transplantation. *Archives of Internal Medicine* 1990; 150:523–527.

Skegg DCG. Multiple sclerosis: nature or nurture: *British Medical Journal* 1991; 302:247–248.

Soloway HB. Patient-initiated laboratory testing: applauding the inevitable. *Journal of the American Medical Association* 1990; 264:1718–1719.

Starzl TE, Fung J, Jordan M, et al. Kidney transplantation under FK 506. *Journal of the American Medical Association* 1990; 264:63–67.

Steinberg D, Parthasarathy S, Carew TE, et al. Beyond cholesterol: modifications of low-density lipoprotein that increase its atherogenicity. *New England Journal of Medicine* 1989; 320(14):915–924.

Steinman L. The development of rational strategies for selective immunotherapy against autoimmune demyelinating disease. *Advances in Immunology* 1991; 49:357–379.

Sternberg H, Segall PE, Waitz H, Ben-Abraham A. Interventive gerontology, cloning and cryonics: relevance to life extension. In *Biomedical Advances in Aging*. New York (1990), Plenum Press, 207–219.

Szelenyi I. Tomorrow's asthma therapy—are antiasthmatics in the nineties anti-inflammatory drugs? *Agents and Actions* 1991; 32:25–33.

Te Meerman GJ, Dankert-Roelse JE. Pros and cons of neonatal screening for cystic fibrosis. *Advances in Experimental Medicine and Biology* 1991; 290:83–95.

Thoburn R. Rheumatology at a crossroad. *Journal of Rheumatology* 1990; 17:577–578.

Tsui L-C, Rommens J, Kerem B, et al. Molecular genetics of cystic fibrosis. *Advances in Experimental Medicine and Biology* 1991; 290:9–18.

Van Tol HHM, Bunzow JR, Guan HC. Cloning of the gene for a human dopamine $D_4$ receptor with high affinity for the antipsychotic clozapine. *Nature* 1991; 350:610–614.

Verma I. Gene therapy. *Scientific American* 1990; November:68–84.

Wachter R. AIDS, activism and the politics of health. *New England Journal of Medicine* 1992; 326(2):128–132.

Wainwright B. The molecular pathology of cystic fibrosis. *Currents in Biology* 1991; 1:80–82.

Weisburger J. Nutritional approach to cancer prevention with emphasis on vitamins, antioxidants and carotenoids. *American Journal of Clinical Nutrition* 1991; 53:226S–237S.

White MB, Amos J, Hsu JMC, et al.   A frame-shift mutation in the cystic fibrosis gene. *Nature* 1990; 334:665–667.

Wight JP.   Ethics, commerce and kidneys. *British Medical Journal* 1991; 303:110.

Wilfond BS, Fost N.   The cystic fibrosis gene: medical and social implications for heterozygote detection. *Journal of the American Medical Association* 1990; 263:2777–2783.

Williamson R.   The identification of the CF (cystic fibrosis) gene. Recent progress and new research strategies. Cystic fibrosis—a strategy for the future. *Advances in Experimental Medicine and Biology* 1991; 290:1–7.

World Health Organization.   Special programme of research, development and research training in human reproduction. *Biennial Report 1988–1989.*

Ziff M.   Rheumatoid arthritis—its present and future. *Journal of Rheumatology* 1990; 17(2):127–133.

Ziff, M.   Role of endothelium in chronic inflammation. *Springer Seminars in Immunopathology* 1989; 11:199–214.

Zivin JA, Choi DW. Stroke therapy. *Scientific American* 1991; July:56–63.

--------- CHAPTER 6: THE CONQUEST OF CANCER ---------

Baker SJ, Fearon ER, Nigro JM, et al.   Chromosome 17 deletions and p53 gene mutations in colorectal carcinomas. *Science* 1989; 244:217–221.

Balkwill FRM, Naylor S, Malik S.   Tumor necrosis factor as an anticancer agent. *European Journal of Cancer* 1990; 26(5):641–644.

Baum M, Ziv Y, Colletta A.   Prospects for the chemoprevention of breast cancer. *British Medical Bulletin* 1991; 47(2):493–503.

Bishop JM.   Cancer genes come of age. *Cell* 1983; 32:1018–1020.

Bonney GE.   Interactions of genes, environment and life-style in lung cancer development. *Journal of the National Cancer Institute* 1990; 82:1236–1237.

Bourne HR.   Consider the coiled coil. *Nature* 1991; 351:188–189.

Busch H.   The final common pathway of cancer. *Cancer Research* 1990; 50:4830–4838.

Caparoso NE, Tucker MA, Hoover RN, et al.   Lung cancer and the debrisoquine metabolic phenotype. *Journal of the National Cancer Institute* 1990; 82:1264–1272.

Cavenee WK.   Recessive mutations in the causation of human cancer. *Cancer* 1991; 67:2431–2435.

Chen P-L, Chen Y, Bookstein R, Wen-Hwa L.   Genetic mechanisms of tumor suppression by the human p53 gene. *Science* 1990; 250:1576–1580.

Cipra BA. Cancer vaccines show promise at last. *Science* 1989; 245:813–814.

Clayson DB. Introduction: an overview of current and anticipated methods for cancer prevention. *Cancer Letters* 1990; 50:3–9.

Coles C, Thompson AM, Elder PA, et al. Evidence implicating at least two genes on chromosome 17p in breast carcinogenesis. *Lancet* 1990; 336:761–763.

Cossman J, Schlegel R. p53 in the diagnosis of human neoplasia. *Journal of the National Cancer Institute* 1991; 83(14):980–981.

Culliton BJ. Gene therapy: into the home stretch. *Science* 1990; 249:974–976.

Dulbecco R. A turning point in cancer research: sequencing the human genome. *Science* 1986; 231:1055–1056.

Fearon E, et al. Identification of a chromosome 18q gene that is altered in colorectal carcinoma. *Science* 1990; 247:49–56.

Fidler IJ. Host and tumour factors in cancer metastasis. *European Journal of Clinical Investigation* 1990; 20:481–486.

Floyd RA. Role of oxygen free radicals in carcinogenesis and brain ischemia. *Federation of American Societies for Experimental Biology Journal* 1990; 4:2587–2598.

Gatanga T, Lentz R, Masunaka I, et al. Identification of TNF-LT blocking factor(s) in the serum and ultrafiltrates of human cancer patients. *Lymphokine Research* 1990; 9(2):225–229.

Goldenberg D. Challenges to the therapy of cancer with monoclonal antibodies. *Journal of the National Cancer Institute* 1991; 83(2):78–79.

Greaves MW. The new dermatology. *British Medical Journal* 1990; 300:413–414.

Greenway HT, Cornell RC. Interferon: coming of age. *Archives of Dermatology* 1990; 126:1080–1082.

Gullick WJ. New developments in the molecular biology of breast cancer. *European Journal of Cancer* 1990; 26(4):509–510.

Hollingsworth RE, Wen-Hwa L. Tumor suppressor genes: new prospects for cancer research. *Journal of the National Cancer Institute* 1991; 83:91–96.

Hollstein M, Sidransky D, Vogelstein B, Harris CC. p53 mutations in human cancers. *Science* 1991; 253:49–53.

Hsu IC, Metcalf RA, Sun T, et al. Mutational hotspot in the p53 gene in human hepatocellular carcinomas. *Nature* 1991; 350:427–428.

Huang HJ, Lee JK, Shew JY, et al. Suppression of the neoplastic phenotype by replacement of the RB gene in human cancer cells. *Science* 1988; 242:1563–1566.

Kaidbey KH. The photoprotective potential of the new superpotent sunscreens. *Journal of the American Academy of Dermatology* 1990; 22:449–452.

Kinnon C, Levinsky RJ. Gene therapy for cancer. *European Journal of Cancer* 1990; 26(5):638–640.

Lee JAH. The melanoma epidemic thus far. *Mayo Clinic Proceedings* 1990; 65:1368–1371.

Malkin D, Li FP, Strong LC, et al. Germ line p53 mutations in a familial syndrome of breast cancer, sarcomas and other neoplasms. *Science* 1990; 250:1233–1238.

Marx J. Gene identified for inherited cancer susceptibility. *Science* 1991; 253(5020):616.

Marx J. New clue to cancer metastasis found. *Science* 1990; 249:482–483.

Marx, J. Oncogenes evoke new cancer therapies. *Science* 1990; 249:1376–1378.

Marx, J. Possible new colon cancer gene found. *Science* 1991; vol. 253: 1317.

Marx J. Zeroing in on individual cancer risk. *Science* 1991; 253(5020):612–616.

Meyskens FL. Coming of age—the chemoprevention of cancer. *New England Journal of Medicine* 1990; 323:825–826.

Moore MAS. The future of cytokine combination therapy. *Cancer* 1991; 67:2718–2726.

Muir CS. Epidemiology, basic science and the prevention of cancer: implications for the future. *Cancer Research* 1990; 50:6441–6448.

Naber SP, Tsutsumi Y, Yin S, et al. Strategies for the analysis of oncogene overexpression. *American Journal of Clinical Pathology* 1990; 94:125–136.

Nigro JM, et al. Mutations in the p53 gene occur in diverse tumor types. *Nature* 1989; 342:705–708.

Nishisho I, Nakamura Y, Miyoshi Y, et al. Mutations of chromosome 5q21 genes in FAP and colorectal cancer patients. *Science* 1991; 253(5020):665–669.

Nowell PC. How many human cancer genes? *Journal of the National Cancer Institute* 1991; 83(15):1061–1064.

Nowell PC. Molecular events in tumor development. *New England Journal of Medicine* 1988; 319:575–577.

Parkinson DR, Abrams JS, Wiernik P, et al. Interleukin-2 therapy in patients with metastatic malignant melanoma: a phase II study. *Journal of Clinical Oncology* 1990; 8:1650–1656.

Pryor WA. The antioxidant nutrients and disease prevention—what do we know and what do we need to find out? *American Journal of Clinical Nutrition* 1991; 53:391S–393S.

Roberts L. Testing for cancer risk: tough questions ahead. *Science* 1991; 253(5020):614–615.

Rosenberg S. Adoptive immunotherapy for cancer. *Scientific American* 1990; May:62–69.

Rosenberg SA., Aebersold P, Cornetta K, et al. Gene transfer into humans—immunotherapy of patients with advanced melanoma, using tumor-infiltrating lymphocytes modified by retroviral gene transduction. *New England Journal of Medicine* 1990; 323:570–578.

Sato T, Kazuhiro Y, et al. Allelotype of breast cancer: cumulative allele losses promote tumor progression in primary breast cancer. *Cancer Research* 1990; 50:7184–7189.

Scanlon EF. Progress in the treatment of early breast cancer. *Cancer* 1990; 65:2110–2112.

Sellers TA, Bailey-Wilson JE, Elston RC, et al. Evidence for mendelian inheritance in the pathogenesis of lung cancer. *Journal of the National Cancer Institute* 1990; 82:1272–1279.

Shields PG, Harris CC. Molecular epidemiology and the genetics of environmental cancer. *Journal of the American Medical Association* 1991; 266:681–687.

Sidransky D, Eschenbach A, Tsai YC, et al. Identification of p53 gene mutations in bladder cancers and urine samples. *Science* 1991; 252:706–709.

Skolnick A. Molecular biology research offers new weapons against cancer. *Journal of the American Medical Association* 1990; 263(17):2289–2290.

Slebos RJC, Kibbelaar R, Dalesio O, et al. K-ras oncogene activation as a prognostic marker in adenocarcinoma of the lung. *New England Journal of Medicine* 1990; 323:561–565.

Stoler AB. Genes and cancer. *British Medical Bulletin* 1991; 47(1):64–75.

Studzinski GP, Moore D, Carter DL. Suppressor genes; restraint of growth or of tumor progression? *Laboratory Investigation* 1990; 63(3):279–282.

Vogelstein B. A deadly inheritance. *Nature* 1990; 348:681–682.

Vogelstein B, et al. Genetic alterations during colorectal-tumor development. *New England Journal of Medicine* 1988; 319:525–532.

Warrell RP, Frankel SR, Wilson M, Jr, et al. Differentiation therapy of acute promyelocytic leukemia with tretinoin (all *trans*-retinoic acid). *New England Journal of Medicine* 1991; 324:1385–1393.

Weinberg R. The genetic origins of human cancer. *Cancer* 1988; 61:1963–1968.

Weisburger J. Nutritional approach to cancer prevention with emphasis on vitamins, antioxidants and carotenoids. *American Journal of Clinical Nutrition* 1991; 53:226S–237S.

Willman C, Fenoglio-Presier CM. Oncogenes, suppressor genes and carcinogenesis. *Human Pathology* 1987; 18(9):895–902.

Yandell DW, Campbell TA, Dayton SH, et al. Oncogene point mutations in the human retinoblastoma gene: their application to genetic counselling. *New England Journal of Medicine* 1989; 321:1689–1695.

Zielinski CC, Mueller C, Tyl E, et al. Impaired production of tumor necrosis factor in breast cancer. *Cancer* 1990; 66:1944–1948.

—————— CHAPTER 7: THE END OF CORONARY DISEASE ——————

Aalto-Setälä K. Molecular genetics of hypercholesterolemia. *Annals of Medicine* 1990; 22:1–2.

Alderman MH, Madhavan S, Ooi WL, et al. Association of the renin-sodium profile with the risk of myocardial infarction in patients with hypertension. *New England Journal of Medicine* 1991; 324:1098–1104.

Austin MA, King M-C, Vranizan KM, Kraus RM. Atherogenic lipoprotein phenotype: a proposed genetic marker for coronary heart disease risk. *Circulation* 1990; 82:495–506.

Berman DS, Kiat H, Van Train KF, et al. Comparison of SPECT using technitium-99m agents and thallium-201 and PET for the assessment of myocardial perfusion and viability. *American Journal of Cardiology* 1990; 66:72E–79E.

Blakeslee S. Common virus seen as having early role in arteries' clogging. *The New York Times, Medical Science*, January 29, 1991.

Bonan R, Bhat K, Lefèvre T, et al. Coronary artery stenting after angioplasty with self-expanding parallel wire metallic stents. *American Heart Journal* 1990; 121(5):1522–1529.

Breslow JL. Genetic basis of lipoprotein disorders. *Journal of Clinical Investigation* 1989; 84:373–380.

Breslow JL. Lipoprotein transport abnormalities underlying coronary heart disease susceptibility *(in press)*.

Cybulsky MI, Gimbrone Ma, Jr. Endothelial expression of a mononuclear leukocyte adhesion molecule during atherogenesis. *Science* 1991; 251:788–791.

Davies SW, Ranjadayalan K, Wickens DC, et al. Lipid peroxidation associated with successful thrombolysis. *Lancet* 1990; 335:741–743.

Dieber-Rothender M, Puhl H, Waeg G, Striegl G, Esterbauer H. Effect of oral supplementation with D-α-tocopherol on the vitamin E content of human low-density lipoproteins and resistance to oxidation. *Journal of Lipid Research* 1991; 32:1325–1332.

Gey KF, Puska P. Plasma vitamins E and A inversely correlated to mortality from ischemic heart disease in cross-cultural epidemiology.

*Annals of the New York Academy of Sciences* 1989; 570:268–282.

Gimbrone MA, Jr, Bevilacqua MP, Cybulsky MI.   Endothelial-dependent mechanisms of leukocyte adhesion in inflammation and atherosclerosis. *Annals of the New York Academy of Sciences* 1990; 410:77–85.

Goldsmith M.   Cold laser, arterial stent studies continue. *Journal of the American Medical Association* 1990; 264(21):2727–2728.

Goy J-J, Sigwart U, Vogt P, et al.   Long-term follow-up of the first 56 patients treated with intracoronary self-expanding stents (the Lausanne experience). *American Journal of Cardiology* 1991; 67:569–572.

Grundy SM.   Cholesterol and coronary heart disease: future directions. *Journal of the American Medical Association* 1990; 264(23):3053–3059.

Haber E.   Can plasminogen activators be improved? *Circulation* 1990; 82(5):1875–1876.

Hansson GK, Jonasson L, Seifert P, Stemme S.   Immune mechanisms in atherosclerosis. *Arteriosclerosis* 1989; 9:567–587.

Holmes DR, Jr, Vlietstra RE, Reiter SJ, Bresnahan DR.   Advances in interventional cardiology. *Mayo Clinic Proceedings* 1990; 65:565–583.

Kennedy JW.   Expanding the use of thrombolytic therapy for acute myocardial infarction. *Annals of Internal Medicine* 1990; 113(12):907–908.

Krauss RM.   The tangled web of coronary risk factors. *American Journal of Medicine* 1991; 90:36S–41S.

Krieger JE, Dzqu VJ.   Molecular biology of hypertension. *Hypertension* 1991; 18(3), supplement:I3–I17.

Kuzuya F, Kuzuya M, Yasue M, et al.   Clinical and experimental approaches to the prevention of atherosclerosis by immunological regulations. *Annals of the New York Academy of Sciences* 1990; 410:459–463.

Lefer A, Tsao P, Aoki N, Palladino MA, Jr.   Mediation of cardioprotection by transforming growth factor-β. *Science* 1990; 249:61–64.

Leger JOC, Larue C, Tao Ming, et al.   Assay of serum cardiac myosin heavy chain fragments in patients with acute myocardial infarction: determination of infarct size and long-term follow-up. *American Heart Journal* 1990; 120:781–790.

Lerman A, Edwards BS, Hallett JW, et al.   Circulating and tissue endothelin immunoreactivity in advanced atherosclerosis. *New England Journal of Medicine* 1991; 325:997–1001.

Litvack F, Eigler NL, Margolis JR, et al.   Percutaneous excimer laser coronary angioplasty. *American Journal of Cardiology* 1990; 66:1027–1032.

Mahley RW, Weisgraber KH, Innerarity TL, Rall SC Jr.   Genetic defects in lipoprotein metabolism. *Journal of the American Medical Association* 1991; 265:78–83.

Masayuki Y, Hammer R, Ishibashi S, Brown MS, Goldstein JL. Diet-induced hypercholesterolemia in mice: prevention by overexpression of LDL receptors. *Science* 1990; 250:1273–1275.

Matsumori A, Yamada T, Tamaki N, et al. Persistent uptake of indium-111-antimyosin monoclonal antibody in patients with myocardial infarction. *American Heart Journal* 1990; 120(5):1026–1030.

McAfee J. Nuclear medicine comes of age: its present and future roles in diagnosis. *Radiology* 1990; 174:609–620.

Muller DWM, Ellis S, Debowey DL, Topol EJ. Quantitative angiographic comparison of the immediate success of coronary angioplasty, coronary atherectomy and endoluminal stenting. *American Journal of Cardiology* 1990; 66:938–942.

Nabel E, Nabel G. Gene transfer and cardiovascular disease. *Trends in Cardiovascular Medicine* (in press).

Nabel E, Plautz G, Boyce FM, et al. Recombinant gene expression in vivo within endothelial cells of the arterial wall. *Science* 1989; 244:1342–1344.

Nabel EG, Plautz G, Nabel G. Site-specific gene expression in vivo by direct gene transfer into the arterial wall. *Science,* (in press).

Nestel PJ. New lipoprotein profiles and coronary heart disease: improving precision of risk. *Circulation* 1990; 82(2):649–650.

Olman EM, Casey C, Bengston J, et al. Early detection of acute myocardial infarction: additional diagnostic information from serum concentrations of myoglobin in patients without ST elevation. *British Heart Journal* 1990; 63:335–338.

Orekhov AN, Tetrov VV, Kabakov AE, et al. Autoantibodies against modified low-density lipoprotein. *Arteriosclerosis and Thrombosis* 1991; 11:316–326.

Palinski W, Rosenfeld ME, Ylä-Herttuala S, et al. Low-density lipoprotein undergoes oxidative modification in vivo. *Proceedings of the National Academy of Sciences USA* 1989; 86:1372–1376.

Palinski W, Ylä-Herttuala S, Rosenfeld ME. Antisera and monoclonal antibodies generated during oxidative modification of low-density lipoprotein. *Arteriosclerosis* 1990; 10:325–335.

Peshock RM. Clinical cardiovascular magnetic resonance imaging. *American Journal of Cardiology* 1990; 66:41F–44F.

Pool R. Making 3-D movies of the heart. *Science* 1991; 251:28–30.

Potkin BN, Bartorelli AL, Gessert J. et al. Coronary artery imaging with intravascular high-frequency ultrasound. *Circulation* 1990; 81:1575–1585.

Prasad K, Lee P, Kalra J. Influence of endothelin on cardiovascular function, oxygen free radicals and blood chemistry. *American Heart Journal* 1991; 121(1):178–187.

Rajavashisth TB, Andalibi A, Territo MC, et al. Induction of endothelial cell expression of granulocyte and macrophage colony-stimulating factors by modified low-density lipoproteins. *Nature* 1990; 344:254–257.

Rau L. Hypertension, endothelium and cardiovascular risk factors. *American Journal of Medicine* 1991; 90, supplement:2A–13S.

Reinhart RA, Gani K, Arndt MT, Broste SK. Apolipoproteins A-1 and B as predictors of angiographically defined coronary artery disease. *Archives of Internal Medicine* 1990; 150:1629–1633.

Ross R, Masuda J, Raines EW, et al. Localization of PDGF-B protein in macrophages in all phases of atherogenesis. *Science* 1990; 248:1009–1012.

Ross R, Masuda J, Raines EW. Cellular interactions, growth factors and smooth muscle proliferation in atherogenesis. *Annals of the New York Academy of Sciences* 1990; 410:102–112.

Rubin EM, Krauss RM, Spangler EA, et al. Inhibition of early atherogenesis in transgenic mice by human apolipoprotein A1. *Nature* 1991: 353(6341):265–267.

Safian RD, Gelbfish JS, Erny RE, et al. Coronary atherectomy: clinical, angiographic and histological findings and observations regarding potential mechanisms. *Circulation* 1990; 82:69–79.

Samani NJ. New developments in renin and hypertension. *British Medical Journal* 1991; 302:981–982.

Serruys PW, Strauss BH, Beatt K, et al. Angiographic follow-up after placement of a self-expanding coronary-artery stent. *New England Journal of Medicine* 1991; 324:13–17.

Sigwart U. Percutaneous transluminal coronary angioplasty: what next? *British Heart Journal* 1990; 63:321–322.

Sniderman A, Silberberg J. Is it time to measure apolipoprotein B? *Arterosclerosis* 1990; 10(5):665–667.

Steinberg D. Antioxidants and atherosclerosis: a current assessment. *Circulation* 1991; 84(3):1420–1425.

Steinberg D, Parthasarathy S, Carew TE, et al. Beyond cholesterol: modifications of low-density lipoprotein that increase its atherogenicity. *New England Journal of Medicine* 1989; 320(14):915–924.

Steinberg D, Witztum JL. Lipoproteins and atherogenesis: current concepts. *Journal of the American Medical Association* 1990; 264(23):3047–3052.

Timmis AD. Early diagnosis of acute myocardial infarction. *British Medical Journal* 1990; 301:941–942.

Van der Wall E, de Roos A, van Voorthuisen Ad E, Bruschke

AVG. Magnetic resonance imaging: a new approach for evaluating coronary artery disease? *American Heart Journal* 1990; 121(4):1203–1220.

Veith FJ, Bakal CW, Cynamon J, et al. Early experience with the smart laser in the treatment of atherosclerotic occlusions. *American Heart Journal* 1990; 121(5):1531–1538.

Ylä-Herttuala S, Palinski W, Rosenfeld ME, et al. Evidence for the presence of oxidatively modified low-density lipoprotein in atherosclerotic lesions of rabbit and man. *Journal of Clinical Investigation* 1989; 84:1086–1095.

## CHAPTER 8: SOLVING THE MYSTERY OF ALZHEIMER'S ——— DISEASE AND OTHER NEUROLOGICAL PROBLEMS ———

Anand R, Wesnes KA. Moclobemide, a reversible MAO inhibitor possesses cognition enhancing effects in humans. *Acta Psychiatrica Scandinavica Supplement* 1990; 82/360:71–72.

Choi DW. Cerebral hypoxia: some new approaches and unanswered questions. *Journal of Neuroscience* 1990; 10(8):2493–2501.

Council on Long Range Planning and Development, American Medical Association. The future of psychiatry. *Journal of the American Medical Association* 1990; 264(19):2542–2548.

Davis RE, Moos WH. Cholinergic replacement in dementia: past and future perspectives. *Clinical Advancements in Alzheimer's Disease, in press.*

DeNoble VJ, DeNoble KF, Spencer KR, et al. Comparison of Dup 996, with physostigmine, THA and 3,4-DAP on hypoxia-induced amnesia in rats. *Pharmacology, Biochemistry and Behavior* 1991; 36:957–961.

Dunnett S. Cholinergic grafts, memory and aging. *Trends in Neurosciences* 1991; 14(8):372–375.

Eagger SA, Levy R, Sahakian BJ. Tacrine in Alzheimer's disease. *Lancet* 1991; 337:987–992.

Erickson D. Love and terror: is a chemical messenger key to treating Alzheimer's? *Scientific American* 1991; April:148–150.

Fahn S. An open trial of high-dosage antioxidants in early Parkinson's disease. *American Journal of Clinical Nutrition* 1991; 53:380S–382S.

Foster AC. Physiology and pathophysiology of excitatory amino acid neurotransmitter systems in relation to Alzheimer's disease. *Advances in Neurology* 51: 1990; Wurtman R, et al. (eds.). New York, Raven Press, 97–101.

Gage FH, Kawaja MD, Fischer LJ. Genetically modified cells: applications for intracerebral grafting. *Trends in Neurosciences* 1991; 14(8):328–333.

Gamzu ER, Thal LJ, Davis KL. Therapeutic trials using tacrine and other cholinesterase inhibitors. In Wurtman R, et al. (eds.). *Advances in Neurology* 51. New York (1990), Raven Press, 241–245.

Goate AM, Hardy JA, Owen MJ, et al. Genetics of Alzheimer's disease. In Wurtman R, et al. (eds.). *Advances in Neurology* 51. New York (1990), Raven Press, 197–198.

Goate AM, Haynes AR, Owen MJ, et al. Predisposing locus for Alzheimer's disease on chromosome 21. *Lancet* 1989; II:352–355.

Golbe LI. The genetics of Parkinson's disease: a reconsideration. *Neurology* 1990; 40(supplement 3):7–14.

Goldgaber D, Schmechel DE. Expression of the amyloid β- protein precursor gene. In Wurtman R, et al. (eds.). *Advances in Neurology* 51. New York (1990), Raven Press, 163–169.

Greeley HT, Hamm T, Johnson R, et al. The ethical use of human fetal tissue in medicine. *New England Journal of Medicine* 1989; 320(16):1093–1096.

Johnson KA, Holman BL, Rosen J, et al. Iofetamine I-123 single photon emission computed tomography is accurate in the diagnosis of Alzheimer's disease. *Archives of Internal Medicine* 1990; 150:752–756.

Jori MC, Franceschi M, Guisti MC, et al. Clinical experience with cabergoline, a new ergoline derivative, in the treatment of Parkinson's disease. *Advances in Neurology* 1990; 53:539–543.

Langston JW. Predicting Parkinson's disease. *Neurology* 1990; 40(supplement 3):70–74.

Langston JW. Selegiline as neuroprotective therapy in Parkinson's disease. *Neurology* 1990; 40(supplement 3):61–66.

Langston JW, Koller WC. The next frontier in Parkinson's disease: presymptomatic detection. *Neurology* 1991; 41(supplement 2):5–7.

Lindvall O. Prospects of transplantation in human neurodegenerative diseases. *Trends in Neurosciences* 1991; 14(8):376–384.

Lowe SL, Bowen DM, Francis PT, Neary D. Ante mortem cerebral amino acid concentrations indicate selective degeneration of glutamate-enriched neurons in Alzheimer's disease. *Neuroscience* 1990; 38(3):571–577.

Marsden CD. Parkinson's disease. *Lancet* 1990; 335:948–952.

Martin GM, Schellenberg GD, Wijsman EM, Bird TD. Alzheimer's disease: dominant susceptibility genes. *Nature* 1990; 347:124.

Marx, J. Alzheimer's pathology explored. *Science* 1990; 249:984–985.

Murrell J, Garlow M, Ghetti B, et al. A mutation in the amyloid precursor protein associated with hereditary Alzheimer's disease. *Science* 1991; 254(5028):97–99.

Oh SM, Betz L. Interaction between free radicals and excitatory amino acids in the formation of ischemic brain edema in rats. *Stroke* 1991; 22:915–921.

Pharmaceutical Manufacturers Association. *Alzheimer's Medicines in Development*, 1989.

Randall T. Alzheimer's-linked protein found to be skin deep, but potential new therapies see beauty of it. *Journal of the American Medical Association* 1991; 265(3)309–310.

St. George-Hyslop PH, Haines JL, Farrer LA, et al. Genetic linkage studies suggest that Alzheimer's disease is not a single homogeneous disorder. *Nature* 1990; 347:194–195.

Schmidley JW. Free radicals in central nervous system ischemia. *Current Concepts of Cerebrovascular Disease and Stroke* 1990; 25:7–12.

Selkoe D. Deciphering Alzheimer's disease: the amyloid precursor protein yields new clues. *Science* 1990; 248:1058–1060.

Snyder SH. Parkinson's disease: fresh factors to consider. *Nature* 1991; 350:195–196.

Tanner CM, Langston JW. Do environmental toxins cause Parkinson's disease? A critical review. *Neurology* 1990; 40(supplement 3):17–30.

Wright AF, Goedert M, Hastie ND. Beta-amyloid resurrected. *Nature* 1991; 349:653–654.

Yanker BA, Mesulam MM. β-Amyloid and the pathogenesis of Alzheimer's disease. *New England Journal of Medicine* 1991; 325(26):1849–1857.

Zivin JA, Choi DW. Stroke therapy. *Scientific American* 1991; July:56–63.

—————————— CHAPTER 9: THE NEXT PLAGUE ——————————

Broder S. (moderator). Antiretroviral therapy in AIDS. *Annals of Internal Medicine* 1990; 113(8):604–618.

Culliton BJ. Gene therapy begins. *Science* 1990; 249:1372.

Kilbourne ED. New viral diseases: a real and potential problem without boundaries. *Journal of the American Medical Association* 1990; 264(1):68–70.

Mitsuya H, Yarochoan R, Broder S. Molecular targets for AIDS therapy. *Science* 1990; 249:1533–1544.

Verma I. Gene therapy. *Scientific American* 1990; November:68–84.

Weatherall DJ. Gene therapy in perspective. *Nature* 1991; 349:275.

— CHAPTER 10: THE FUTURE OF EVERYDAY COMPLAINTS —

Albert MB, Fromm H, Borstelmann R, et al. Successful outpatient treatment of gallstones with piezoelectric lithotripsy. *Annals of Internal Medicine* 1990; 113(2):164–166.

Balin AK, Allen RG. Molecular bases of biologic aging. *Clinics in Geriatric Medicine* 1989; 5(1):1–21.

Bousquet J, Hejjaoui A, Michel FB. Specific immunotherapy in asthma. *Journal of Allergy and Clinical Immunology* 1990; 86(3):292–305.

Bruckstein AH. Nonsurgical management of cholelithiasis. *Archives of Internal Medicine* 1990; 150:960–964.

Bukantz S, Lockey R. Allergy and immunology: Contempo 1991. *Journal of the American Medical Association* 1991; 265(23):3101–3103.

Cady RK, Wendt JK, Kirchner JR, et al. Treatment of acute migraine with subcutaneous sumatriptan. *Journal of the American Medical Association* 1991; 265:2831–2835.

Canalis E, McCarthy TL, Centrella M. Growth factors and cytokines in bone cell metabolism. *Annual Review of Medicine* 1991; 42:17–24.

Catalona WJ, Smith DS, Ratliff TL, et al. Measurement of prostate-specific antigen in serum as a screening test for prostate cancer. *New England Journal of Medicine* 1991; 324:1156–1161.

Christiansen C. Consensus development conference: prophylaxis and treatment of osteoporosis. *American Journal of Medicine* 1991; 90:107–110.

Cotton P. Case for prostate therapy wanes despite more treatment options. *Journal of the American Medical Association* 1991; 266(4):459–460.

Cutler RG. Antioxidants and aging. *American Journal of Clinical Nutrition* 1991; 53:373S–379S.

Editorial. New treatments for osteoporosis. *Lancet* 1990; 335:1065–1066.

Ferluga J. Potential role of anti-oncogenes in aging. *Mechanisms of Aging and Development* 1990; 53:267–275.

Ferrari, MD, et al. (The Subcutaneous Sumatriptan International Study Group). Treatment of migraine attacks with sumatriptan. *New England Journal of Medicine* 1991; 325:316–321.

Geokas MC (moderator). The aging process. *Annals of Internal Medicine* 1990; 113:455–466.

Gibbons A. Gerontology research comes of age. *Science* 1990; 250:622–625.

Goadsby PJ, Zagami AS, Donnan GA. Oral sumatriptan in acute migraine. *Lancet* 1991; 338(8770):782–783.

Goldsmith M.    Future surgery: minimal invasion. *Journal of the American Medical Association* 1990; 262(21):2723.

Goldstein S.    Replicative senescence: the human fibroblast comes of age. *Science* 1990; 249:1129–1133.

Gordon J.    The human genome project promises insight into aging. *Geriatrics* 1989; 44:89–91.

Gostout CJ.    Gastrointestinal laser endoscopy—future horizons. *Mayo Clinic Proceedings* 1990; 65:509–517.

Heaney RP, Avioli LV, Chestnut C III, et al.    Osteoporotic bone fragility: detection by ultrasound transmission velocity. *Journal of the American Medical Association* 1989: 261:2986–2990.

Hoffman AF.    Nonsurgical treatment of gallstone disease. *Annual Review of Medicine* 1990; 41:401–415.

Lerner RA, Benkovic SJ.    Observations in the interface between immunology and chemistry. *Chemtracts—Organic Chemistry* 1990; 3:1–36.

Lerner RA, Benkovic SJ, Schultz PG.    At the crossroads of chemistry and immunology: catalytic antibodies. *Science* 1991; 252:659–667.

Lindsay R.    Managing osteoporosis: current trends, future possibilities. *Geriatrics* 1987; 42(3):35–39.

Maier JAM, Voulalas P, Roeder D, Maciag T.    Extension of the life-span of human endothelial cells by an interleukin-1α antisense oligomer. *Science* 1990; 249:1570–1574.

Olshansky SJ, Carnes BA, Cassel C.    In search of Methuselah: estimating the upper limits to human longevity. *Science* 1990; 250:634–640.

Peck WA, Riggs BL, Bell NH, et al.    Research directions in osteoporosis. *American Journal of Medicine* 1988; 84:275–282.

Raisz LG.    Local and systemic factors in the pathogenesis of osteoporosis. *New England Journal of Medicine* 1988; 318(13):818–828.

Schoenfield LJ, Berci G, Carnovale RL, et al.    The effect of ursodial on the efficacy and safety of extracorporeal shock-wave lithotripsy of gallstones. *New England Journal of Medicine* 1990; 323:1239–1245.

Storm T, Thamsborg G, Steinche T, et al.    Effect of intermittent cyclical etidronate therapy on bone mass and fracture rate in women with postmenopausal osteoporosis. *New England Journal of Medicine* 1990; 322:1265–1271.

——————————— EPILOGUE ———————————

Andrews L, Jaeger A.    Confidentiality of genetic information in the workplace. *American Journal of Law and Medicine* 1991; 17:75–108.

Beck MN.    Eugenic abortion: an ethical critique. *Canadian Medical Association Journal* 1990; 143(3):181–185.

Council on Ethical and Judicial Affairs, American Medical Association. Use of genetic testing by employers. *Journal of the American Medical Association* 1991; 266:1827–1830.

Goston L. Genetic discrimination: the use of genetically based diagnostic and prognostic tests by employers and insurers. *American Journal of Law and Medicine* 1991; 17:109–144.

Kolata G. Genetic screening raises questions for employers and insurers. *Science* 1986; 232:317–319.

Murray TH. Ethical issues in human genome research. *Federation of American Societies for Experimental Biology Journal* 1991; 5:55–60.

Rudman D, Feller AG, Nagraj HS, et al. Effects of human growth hormone in men over 60 years old. *New England Journal of Medicine* 1990; 323:1–6.

# INDEX